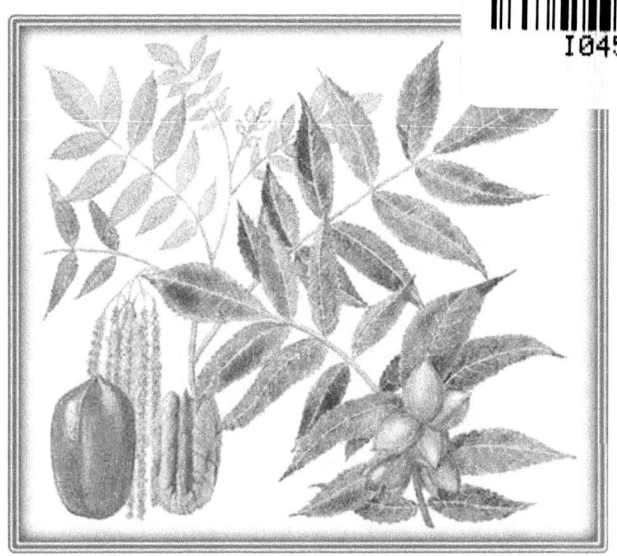

Health Benefits of

Pecans

~by~

James L. Hargrove, Ph.D.

Diane K. Hartle, Ph.D.

Phillip Greenspan, Ph.D.

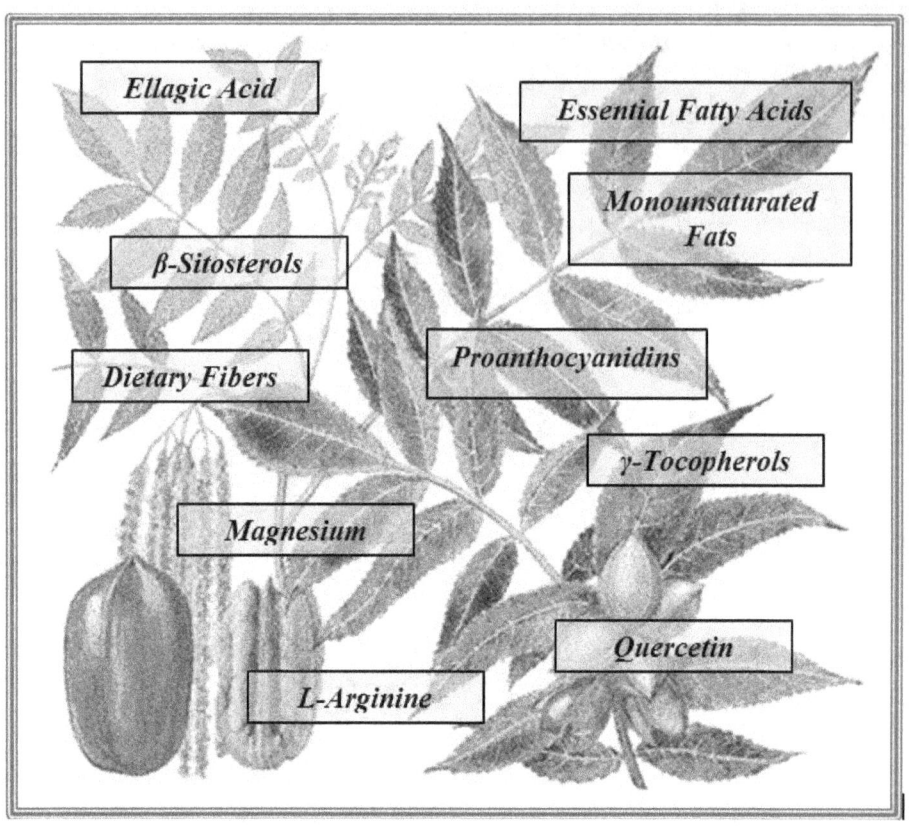

Blue Heron Nutraceuticals, LLC
1180 W. Pine Avenue
St. George Island, FL 32328

ISBN-13: 978-1479318728

© 2013 Blue Heron Nutraceuticals, LLC

Health Benefits of Pecans

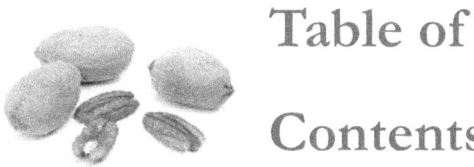

Table of Contents

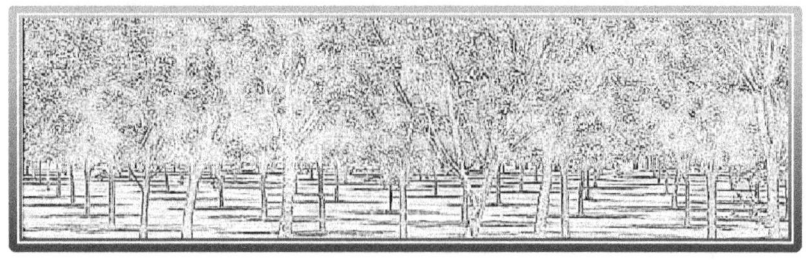

~Caveats~

The views expressed in this book are solely those of the authors after review of pertinent biomedical literature. This book is written for informational purposes on the chemistry and bioactivities of the pecans and pecan products. This book is not a substitute for professional medical advice, diagnosis or treatment of any health condition or problem. Any health care questions regarding your own health should be addressed to your own physician(s) or other health care provider(s). The authors make no warranties nor express or imply representations whatsoever regarding the accuracy, completeness, timeliness, comparative or controversial nature, or usefulness of any information contained or references in this book. Health-related information changes frequently and therefore information contained within this book may be outdated, incomplete or incorrect. Statements made about pecan products have not been evaluated by the Food and Drug Administration. The authors are academic scientists and researchers who engage in nutraceutical research. You are hereby advised to consult with a physician or other professional health-care provider prior to making any decisions, or undertaking any actions or not undertaking any actions related to any health care problem or issue you might have at any time, now or in the future. The authors and Blue Heron Nutraceutical, LLC will not be liable or otherwise responsible for any decision made or any action taken or any action not taken due to your reading of this book

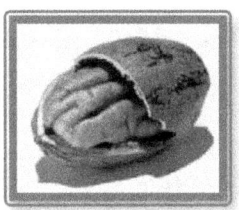

ISBN-13: 978-1479318728

Printed in the United States of America

Pecans and Your Health

What is the Health News about Pecans? The evidence is conclusive: Nuts are good for your family's health. A study of over 30,000 health-conscious Californians showed that people who consumed nuts on a weekly basis gained more than two years of extra life [1].

Especially for adults, the health benefit of nut consumption was impressive; because *it extended life to the same extent as regular exercise.* The study showed that five modest health behaviors could add, on average, **ten years** to people's lifespans. The five behaviors were 1) maintaining a healthy body weight; 2) getting regular, moderate exercise; 3) avoiding cigarette smoking; 4) choosing a diet that is primarily plant-based, and 5) consuming nuts on a weekly basis.

Men and women who consumed nuts and followed these guidelines lived longer because they were less affected by heart disease. Pecans and other nuts are good for heart health when several servings are consumed each week. In the Physicians Health Study, too, the highest level of nut consumption was associated with decreased death from heart disease [2]. Eating nuts helped maintain normal heart rhythm and prevented irregular heartbeats.

Take-Home Message- Including pecans and other nuts in the diet is good for heart health and it increases longevity in men and women. Clearly, nuts contain a treasure trove of beneficial nutrients. This chapter discusses nutritional benefits of pecans and ways that specific phytonutrients in nuts may improve health. There is more good news: small serving sizes provide a great benefit.

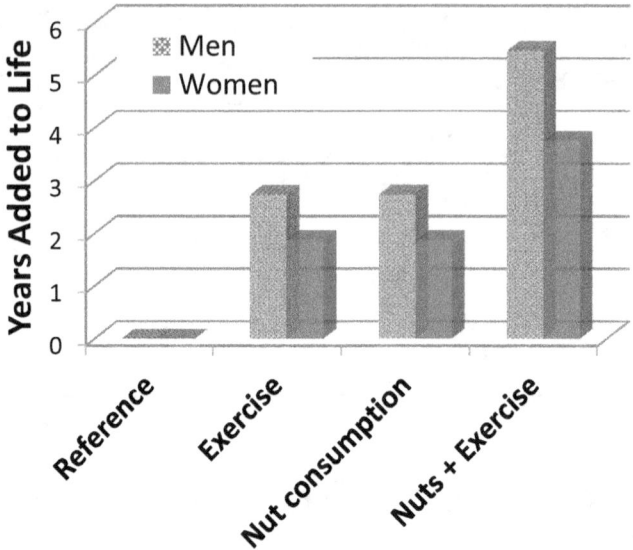

Figure 1.1. **Regular nut consumption and moderate exercise both increased life expectancy for California men (light gray bars) and women (darker bars).** Together, the effects increased lifespan by three years in women and five years in men. Reference group ate nuts less than once per week and did not exercise.

Nuts May Add Years to Your Life- In the California study [1], men who consumed nuts five or more times per week added 2.7 years to their lifespan compared to men who ate nuts no more than once per week. Women who ate nuts at least five times per week gained 1.8 years. *Nut consumption was as effective as regular physical activity* (see **Figure 1.1**).

The benefits of nut consumption are greatest for reducing heart disease. This kind of evidence led the Food and Drug Administration to authorize a qualified health claim for pecans and other nuts, as follows:

FDA Qualified Health Claim for Tree Nuts
Scientific evidence suggests but does not prove that eating 1.5 ounces per day of most nuts, as part of a diet low in saturated fat and cholesterol, may reduce the risk of heart disease.

These facts alone should encourage us to keep nuts handy for snacks and inclusion with breakfast cereals, in salads, entrees, and vegetable side dishes.

What is a Serving of Pecans?   Health benefits of nuts are probably due to improved nutrition of the total diet [3]. The FDA allowed a health claim for improved heart health based on consumption of 1.5 ounces (42 grams (g)) of nuts per day, which is the amount used in the **DASH eating plan** (Dietary Approaches to Stop Hypertension) to lower blood pressure [4]. However, the **serving size for nuts used in dietary planning is one ounce** (28 grams), as shown in the Nutrition Facts panel for pecans shown below. That is about 18 pecan kernels. It is much easier to count pecan halves than to figure weight in ounces. Note that the California study did not measure serving size, it only asked how frequently nuts were consumed.

Pecan Nutrition in a Nutshell- By happy coincidence, the first three letters of NUTrition are "nut." Eating pecans several times each week improves health two ways; first, by providing a nutritionally balanced whole food, and secondly, by displacing snacks that are not well balanced, whole foods. So, what healthful nutrients are we getting each time we eat pecans?

Nutrition Facts

Serving Size 1 ounce (28g)

Amount Per Serving

Calories 193	Calories from Fat 169

	% Daily Value*
Total Fat 20g	31%
Saturated Fat 2g	9%
Trans Fat	
Cholesterol 0mg	0%
Sodium 0mg	0%
Total Carbohydrate 4g	1%
Dietary Fiber 3g	11%
Sugars 1g	
Protein 3g	

Vitamin A	0%	•	Vitamin C	1%
Calcium	2%	•	Iron	4%

*Percent Daily Values are based on a 2,000 calorie diet. Your daily values may be higher or lower depending on your calorie needs.

Pecans are premier sources of healthful monounsaturated fats (12 g per serving) and poly-unsaturated fats (6 g per serving). A serving contains less than 2 g of saturated fats compared to 18 grams of healthful fats.

Pecans are a good source of essential omega-6 fatty acids. They do contain some omega-3 fatty acids.

Whether eaten raw or toasted, pecans contain no cholesterol, no *trans* fats, and no sodium. Pecans are good sources of potassium, which is also beneficial for heart health and blood pressure according to the DASH Eating Plan.

Pecans not only lack cholesterol, they contain compounds that block cholesterol absorption. These cholesterol blockers are called plant sterols, and are waxy substances that prevent cholesterol absorption from the small intestine and uptake into the bloodstream. When cholesterol is not absorbed, it is eliminated from the body, helping to lower cholesterol in the blood plasma. Unlike cholesterol, plant sterols at normal levels of consumption have no adverse effects.

Pecans contain virtually no simple sugars and only a small amount of starch. A one ounce serving also contains 3 g of good quality protein, making pecans an appropriate choice for people who prefer diets with reduced carbohydrate levels and prefer foods with a low glycemic index.

Among all nuts, pecans have some of the highest levels of antioxidants [5-7]. They are rich in the fat-soluble vitamin E family and the vitamin E relative called gamma-tocopherol. They also contain high levels of the plant antioxidant family called polyphenols. Chapter 2 explains this in more depth.

Pecans also contain a number of essential minerals that aid in metabolism. They are good sources of iron and also provide calcium, magnesium and manganese. Iron helps prevent iron-deficiency anemia, and other trace minerals help maintain normal blood pressure and natural antioxidant defenses.

Ten percent of a pecan is dietary fiber that is important for normal cholesterol metabolism and health of the small and large intestines. One serving provides 10% of daily recommended intakes for adults. Most of the fiber in nuts is insoluble, although pecans contain some soluble fiber [8], and nut fiber is thought to help control cholesterol and the glycemic response [9]

Pecans are a low-carbohydrate food and contain very little starch, whether digestible or resistant to digestion. Pecans do contain a variety of non-starch polysaccharides, some of which can be fermented in the large intestine to produce a variety of phytoestrogens called enterolignans [10], which may have health benefits for normal colon health and for prevention of heart disease and some cancers.

Pecans also contain lecithin and other minor lipids that help repair cell membranes, for example nerve cell membranes to maintain good brain health.

The 100 Calorie Snack- Eating pecans several times each week improves health. The effect is largest if pecans are substituted for less nutritious foods or snacks. It is very useful to think in terms of the amount of a food that provides 100 calories, as shown for pecan kernels in **Figure 1.2.**

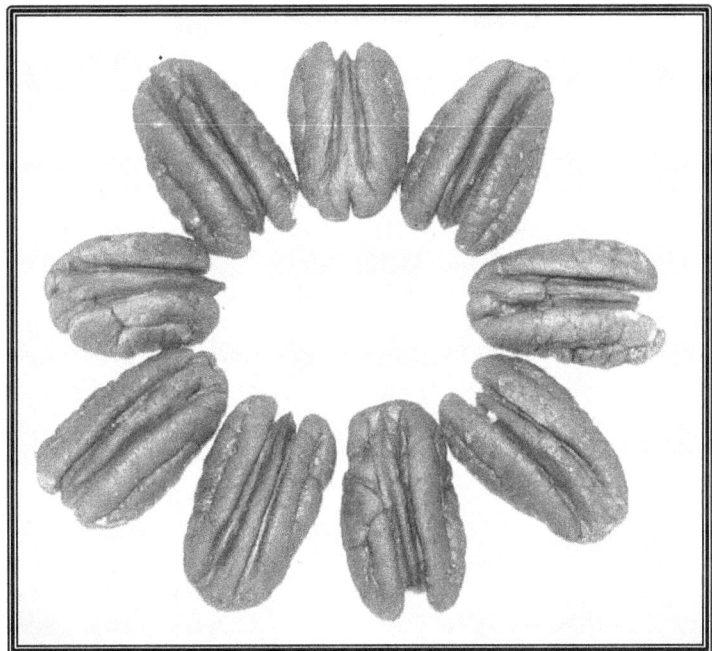

Figure 1.2. A 100 calorie serving of pecan halves is about 9 pieces. A whole pecan kernel before shelling contains two of these pieces. To be consistent, we will consistently refer to these familiar halves as kernels.

In practice, a small handful of nuts (9 or 10 kernels) is a serving. Health benefits can be expected with this amount per day, and more than 2 ounces is unlikely to add any further benefit.

Each shelled nut is actually half of the intact kernel in a whole nut, for clarity, we will refer to a pecan kernel as the familiar shelled kind shown in **Figure 1.2**. Nine shelled pecan kernels contain a total of 100 calories (keeping in mind that the calorie on Nutrition Facts labels is also called a kilocalorie or kcal—don't blame us for the confusion!)

This is useful information because a healthy US man needs about 100 calories an hour averaged over 24 hours a day. For adult US women, the value is closer to 75 calories an hour. For snacking purposes, it is easy to remember that nine kernels will provide a man with the energy he needs for the next hour, and six or seven would suffice for a woman.

Pecans as Low-Glycemic Snacks- The low carbohydrate content of pecans means that they do not raise blood sugar after a meal. Even better, nuts eaten with a meal <u>lower</u> the glycemic effect of the meal! This contrasts with many common snacks found in vending machines. Keeping blood sugar in the normal range is an important part of weight management and reduces the tendency to develop metabolic syndrome or diabetes as an adult.

Pecan Parts-Anatomy of Health- When you eat a pecan, you are eating a whole food, the nutmeat of an American tree. The most powerful phenolic antioxidants in pecans are concentrated in the brown seed coat, which corresponds to the bran of cereal grains. There are lots of commercial varieties of pecans, and some are lighter or darker in color than others. The white nutmeat is the seed itself, but the mixture of contributing phytochemicals differs in these two parts. In nature, the role of the seed is to produce new trees, so it also must be protected against destruction so it can sprout. The antioxidants in the seed coat act as natural sunscreens, ward off insects, and prevent infection by viruses, bacteria and molds. In this case, what is good for the nut also seems to be good for people who eat nuts regularly.

The Nut, Seed and Legume Food Group- Typical US food guides do not have a specific place for nuts, which are usually lumped with seeds and legumes as a source of protein in the Meat group. This is unfortunate because of the important health benefits of nuts.

Several important food guides do list nuts, seeds and legumes as a separate category that should be consumed several times a week. Also, many traditional cuisines consider these to be staple foods that should be eaten on a daily basis. Examples include the Mediterranean Food Guide from Oldways, the evidence-based Harvard Nutrition Source and DASH Eating Plan, and Dr. Weil's Anti-Inflammatory Pyramid.

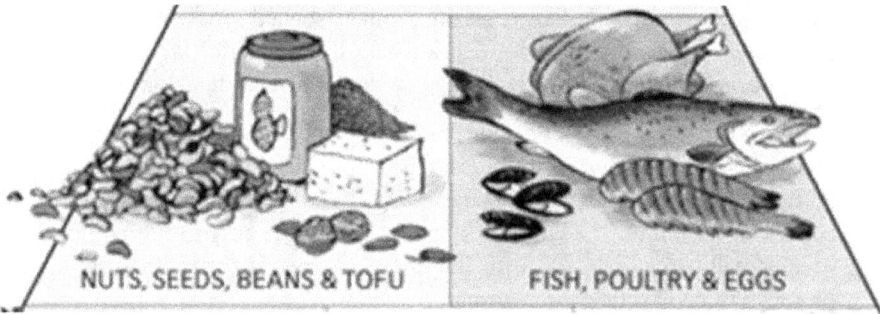

Figure 1.3. Several food guides include a specific category for nuts, nut butters, seeds, beans and soy products. The image above is recommended by the Harvard Nutrition Source.

Pecan Oil and Pecan Butters Until recently, pecan oil has been used as massage oil or incorporated into bath soaps. Compared to commonly used oils like soybean, peanut or olive, pecan oil has a light color and flavor and less saturated fat. As cooking oil, it can be used in salad dressings and other applications. The total content of mono- and polyunsaturated fats in pecan oil is about 90 percent. That is higher than soybean, corn, peanut or canola oils.

Pecan butter is simply made from finely ground pecans. As with any nut butter, the nutrient composition of the nut butter is the same as the original nut. Studies consistently show that nut butters have similar health benefits to whole nuts. In the diet, nut butters are best categorized as **healthful fats**.

What About Nut Allergies? A small proportion of US adults and children develop tree nut allergies, and a person who is allergic to one kind of nut can be allergic to others. Peanut allergies are most common, and affect about one child in 50. However, peanuts are ground nuts (not tree nuts). They are legumes and belong to the bean and pea family. There is no obvious reason that a child with peanut allergies would be allergic to pecans and other tree nuts.

Often, childhood allergies lessen in adulthood. Signs of an allergy may include skin rash or hives, swelling of the joints, shortness of breath, or abdominal pain. If you or your child experiences these signs after eating either tree nuts or ground nuts, the best guidance is to see a physician and avoid nuts and nut products if an allergy is diagnosed.

Biomedical Interest in Pecans and Health- For years, very few medical studies had been done on possible health effects of nuts. This changed when large studies began to associate nut consumption with total health in the early 1990's (**Figure 1.4**). There are now hundreds of studies that concern nuts and health, with new information coming out each month. Medical opinion has shifted to recognize nuts in general and pecans in particular as being excellent whole foods that provide good balance to a complete, healthful diet.

The following chapters will explain recent medical evidence about how and why pecans are good for health. Published studies now show benefits for heart health and blood pressure, for helping to maintain body weight and prevent diabetes, for fighting inflammatory disorders, and for maintaining brain health. The individual effects add up to better chances for a longer, happier life.

With hundreds of scientific publications to choose from, there is a lot to say about pecans and health. Let's get cracking!

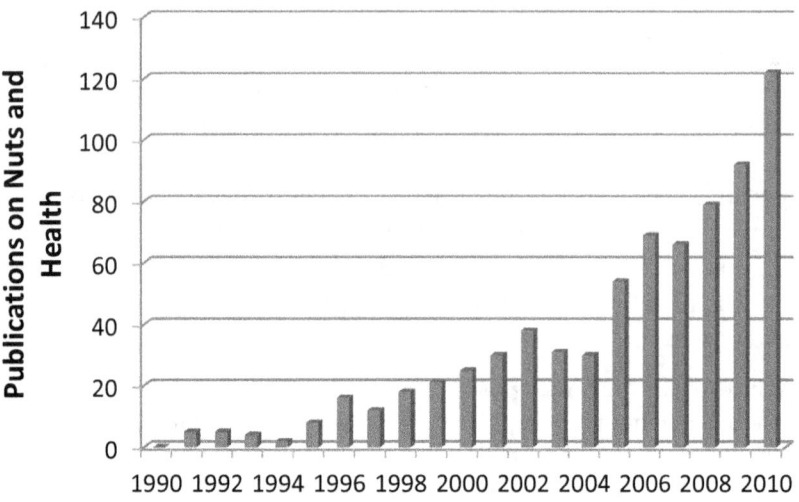

Figure 1.4. Scientific studies on health benefits of nuts are increasing every year. Data were compiled from the PubMed database for the years shown.

Web Resources for Pecan Research and Recipe Ideas

Loma Linda University nut nutrition bibliography

http://www.nutstudies.org/search.php

US Department of Agriculture Nutrient Data Laboratory

http://ndb.nal.usda.gov/

Texas Pecan Board (**includes pecan recipes**)

http://www.texaspecans.org/

Georgia Pecan Commission (**includes pecan recipes**)

http://www.georgiapecans.org/

NutHealth.Org (**includes pecan recipes**)

http://www.nuthealth.org/

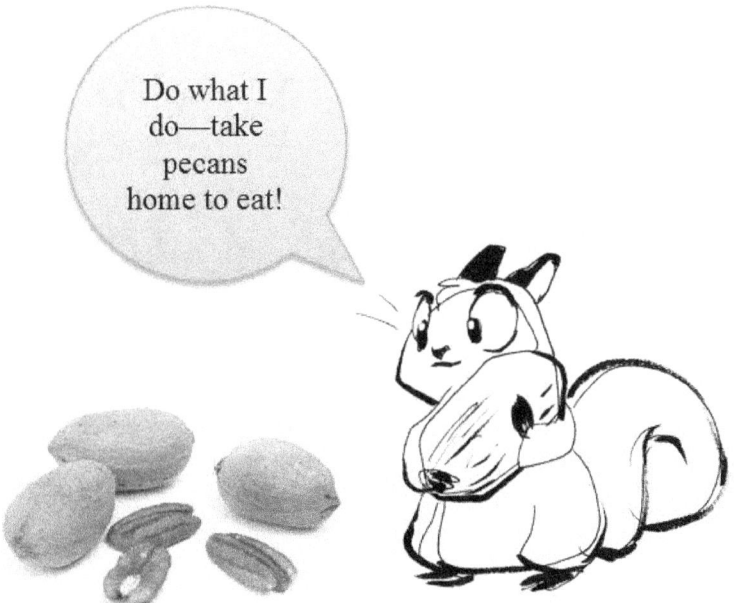

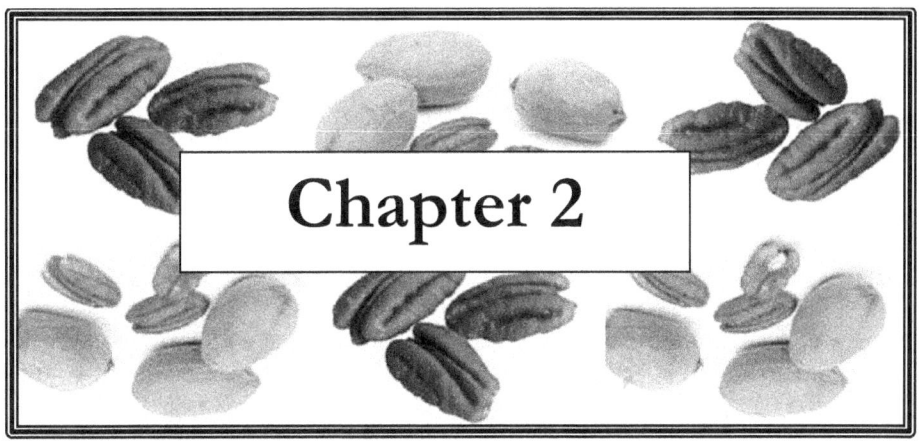

Pecan Antioxidant Power

& Pecan Phytochemicals

Pecan Antioxidant Phytochemicals- Chapter 1 introduced the pecan as a valuable source of essential nutrients including healthy oils, proteins, antioxidant vitamins and minerals in a low-carbohydrate, whole food. In addition to essential nutrients, pecans and other plant-based foods contain an intriguing group of phytochemicals (substances made in plants but not in animals). Many phytochemicals modify our metabolism and help defend our bodies against several common diseases.

A number of families of "plant bioactives" are shown in **Figure 2.1** (next page). Just as human families have numerous related members, every phytochemical family has many chemically related members. Fortunately, it is not necessary to understand all this chemistry to take advantage of pecan phytochemicals in a high quality diet.

Now compare Figure 2.1 with **Figure 2.2**, which shows some specific foods in which specific phytochemicals are abundant. Carotenoids for health of the eye and skin are abundant in orange, red and yellow vegetables such as carrots, squash, and also in dark green leafy vegetables and peppers. Cancer-fighting sulfur compounds are abundant in onions, garlic, cabbage, broccoli and other crucifers.

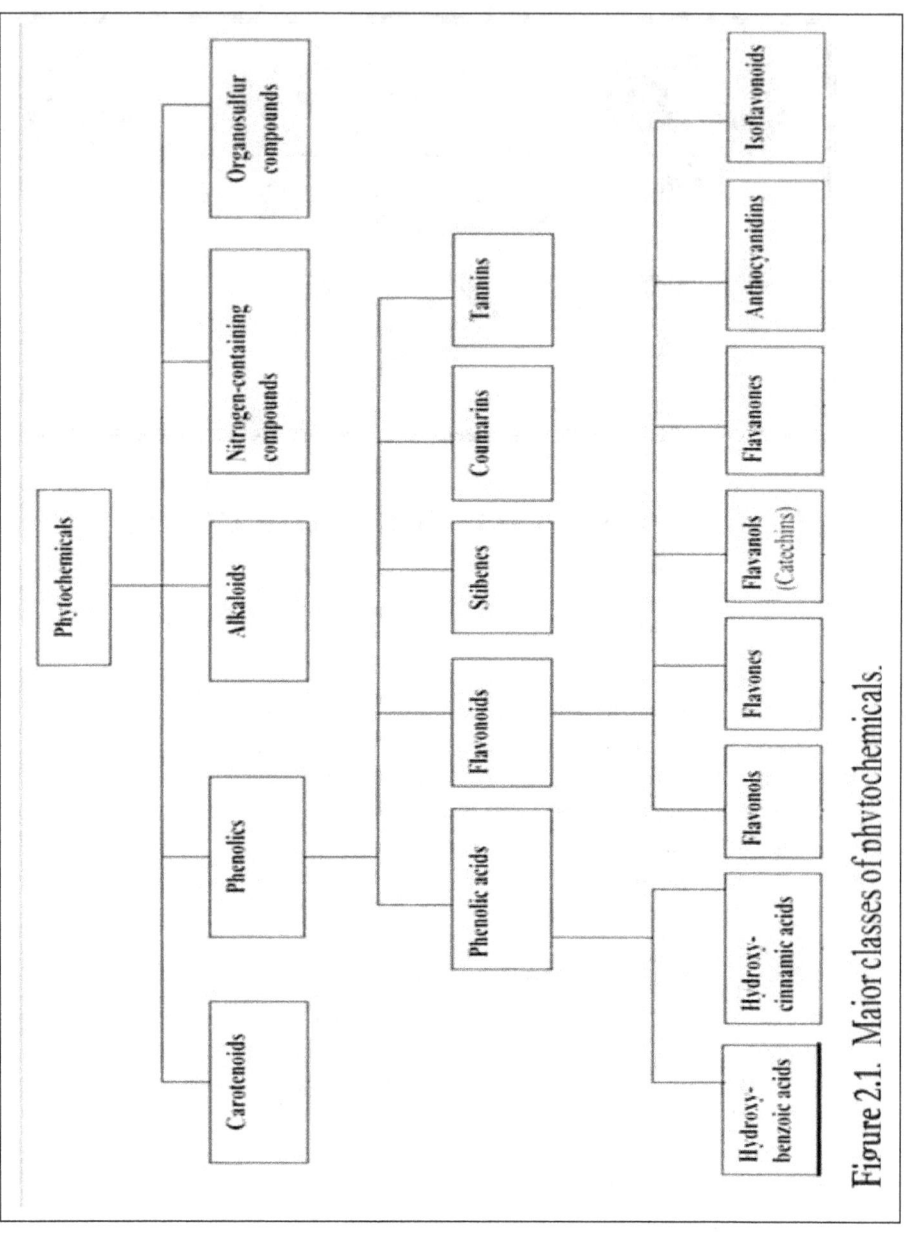

Figure 2.1. Major classes of phytochemicals.

Pecans contain catechins and procyanidins that promote antioxidant defenses and health of the heart, blood vessels and immune system. To improve health, foods containing each of these phytochemical classes should be eaten several times a week in dishes that are full of color and taste.

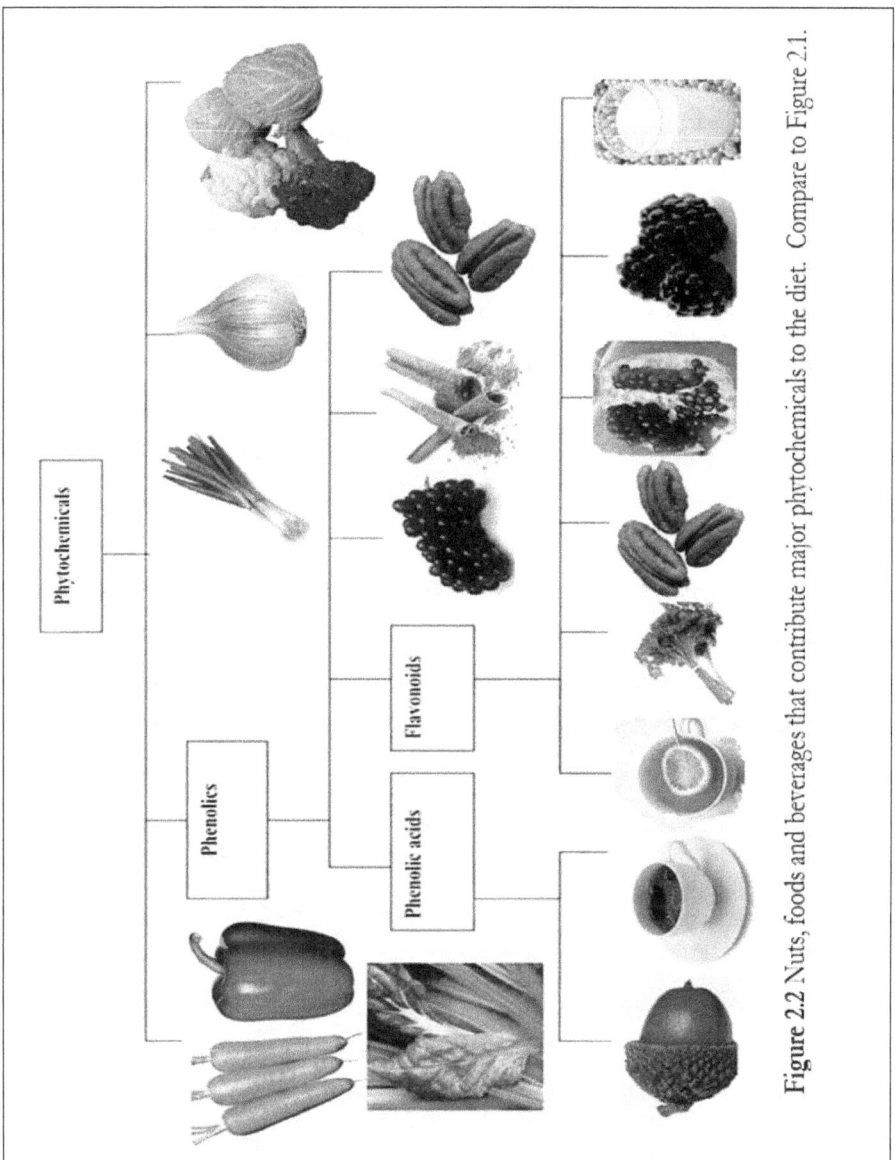

Figure 2.2 Nuts, foods and beverages that contribute major phytochemicals to the diet. Compare to Figure 2.1.

This chapter will explain ways pecans boost diet quality and add to this picture of health.

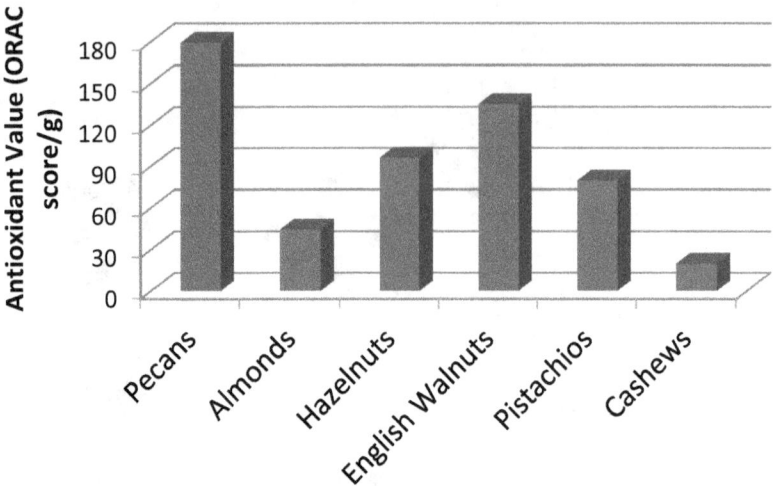

Figure 2.3. Antioxidant value of the main commercial nuts grown in the United States. By several measures, pecans have the highest antioxidant content, even greater than the levels for walnuts [7].

The Body's Antioxidant Defense System- The major cellular antioxidant in the body is called **glutathione**, a compound made from three amino acids (glutamate, cysteine and glycine). If glutathione is maintained at a high level, less vitamins C and E are needed. Conversely, if glutathione levels are depleted, so will vitamins C and E be depleted. Plant polyphenols (such pecan flavonoids) not only preserve existing glutathione but can increase the synthesis of new glutathione in tissues such as muscle and brain. This means that small amounts of polyphenolics can improve antioxidant defenses both directly and indirectly. Polyphenols activate a gene that produces an enzyme that makes glutathione [11, 12]. Pecans have the right polyphenols to provide protection against free radicals in many ways.

The body has mechanisms that are designed to manage normal oxidative stress as best it can. Enzymes such as superoxide dismutase, glutathione peroxidase and glutathione-S-transferases neutralize free radicals and protect against damage caused by free radicals. As part of adaptation to changing needs, our genes direct the production of these enzymes every day. The balance between oxidative stress and antioxidant status is largely the result of gene expression for these defensive enzymes. Pecans and other whole foods in the diet help balance and support these natural defenses.

While the body has its own antioxidant defenses, it is also highly dependent upon the ingestion of antioxidants it cannot produce itself. These come from dietary sources, i.e., food and food supplements. The body needs vitamins C, E and beta-carotene (a precursor of vitamin A). It also needs small amounts of selenium. In addition, the antioxidant defenses of the body are dependent upon various phytochemicals to provide protection in all cells and extracellular spaces in the body. Phytophenolics in pecans provide a broad range of substances that are very important for daily antioxidant support because they not only quench oxidative free radicals, but they enhance the production of the body's own antioxidant defense mechanisms.

How Do Scientists Estimate Antioxidant Power? Three common tests used to evaluate and compare antioxidant values are the **ORAC, FRAP** and **TEAC** assays. ORAC is the Oxygen Radical Absorbance Capacity assay. FRAP is the Ferric Reducing Ability of Plasma assay. TEAC is the Trolox Equivalent Antioxidant Capacity assay. It is important for the consumer to realize that these are simply estimations of antioxidant potential as it can be demonstrated in the laboratory. They are different tests and have different unit values and these units cannot be mixed and matched. An excellent paper was written that compared the ORAC, FRAP and TEAC assays on phenolic extracts of fruits and vegetables, as well as Vitamin C. [13] The study showed that using each assay, there was a direct correlation between ORAC, FRAP and TEAC units and the phenolic fractions tested. Each of these tests is valid for the phytochemistry of the pecan. ORAC values are usually given as micromoles of Trolox (a vitamin E-like antioxidant) equivalents per gram of a solid or per ml of liquid. The higher the number, the greater is the antioxidant power of product.

Remember that these tests simply indicate the total antioxidant activity of a whole mixture of substances in a test tube. The tests do not tell you which substances are contributing to that value, or which is a healthier food. Analytical studies are needed to account for the amount of each phytochemical and its antioxidant contribution. This is not done regularly on commercial products. Most often, the consumer only sees an ORAC score on the whole product. Many laboratories separate out the total phenolic fraction versus the Vitamin C content or may further characterize the phenolic fraction. **Table 2.1** compares the high levels of antioxidants (ORAC values) in pecans with other high antioxidant foods.

In a large survey of common foods, pecans are ranked as the highest antioxidant nut based on Oxygen Radical Absorbance Capacity [6]. Values for

Table 2.1. Highest Antioxidant Activities in Common US Foods and Spices. Data from Wu et al., J. Agric. Food. Chem. **2004**, *52,* 4026-4037.

Whole Food or Spice	Antioxidant Content TE* (μmol per gram)
Cinnamon, ground	2640
Oregano leaf, dried	1831
Cloves, ground	1533
Chocolate, baking	1039
Parsley, dried	740
Basil leaf, dried	644
Turmeric powder	399
Mustard seed, ground	288
Curry powder	249
Chili powder	218
Pecans	**179**
Paprika	161
Walnuts, English	135
Cranberries	94
Blueberries	62
Blackberries	53
Raspberries	49
Bran cereal	25
Whole grain cereal	13

*TE, Trolox equivalents (basis for ORAC assay).

all whole foods depend on many variables related to growing conditions, storage, processing, and analytical methods. Walnuts are close behind pecans in antioxidant content, and both kinds of nut are very healthful when up to one serving is consumed most days of the week. What a great way to snack!

In **Table 2.1**, note that spices and herbs have the highest antioxidant power by any measure. Herbs and spices are not foods in the usual sense. They are very concentrated sources of antioxidants, and are eaten with foods to improve taste. *Pecans and walnuts, along with dark chocolate, berries and cereal bran or whole grain cereals, are actual whole foods that are top antioxidant powerhouses.* Not shown are the thousands of other foods, most of which have much lower antioxidant content than the spices, herbs and foods listed.

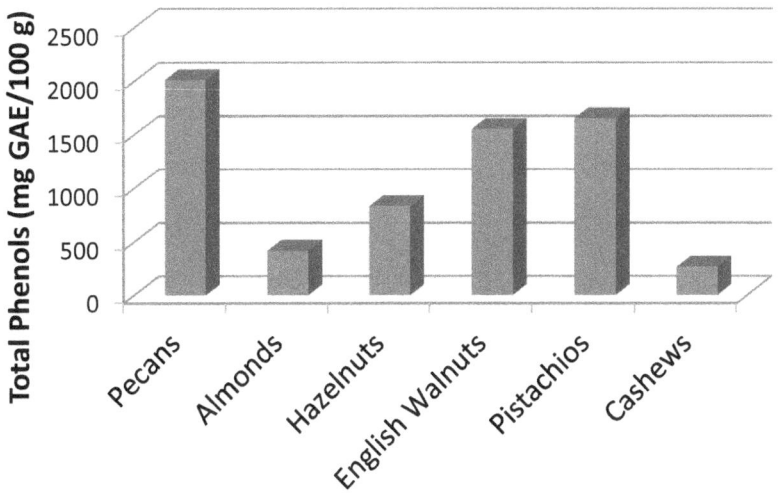

Figure 2.4. Pecans contain the most antioxidant, phenolic compounds among nuts. There is a high correlation between this measurement and antioxidant activity. Data from [7].

Total Phenolic Content of Pecan Products- Many scientists think that the disease-fighting benefits of fruits and berries are only partially due to their ability to provide antioxidant protection. **Figure 2.4** shows that pecans have the greatest amount of phenolics among nuts. It is also very likely that the families of phenolic compounds shown in **Figure 2.1**, which include flavonoids, isoflavones, and stilbenes such as resveratrol, produce specific responses such as reducing inflammation and improving health of the heart and other organs.

No single food item contains all these families of phytochemicals. Pecans do not taste like broccoli or garlic, do they? The key concept is to eat an interesting variety of foods and drink beverages that are rich sources of these compounds on a daily basis, according to each person's taste preferences.

Pecan Antioxidant Power- The typical American consumes only 2-3 servings of fruit and vegetables per day, yielding about 5,700 units of total antioxidant power as measured by the ORAC test [6]. One ounce of pecans (28 grams) contains about 5,000 units of antioxidant power. *The 1.5 ounce serving used for nuts in the DASH eating plan generates 7,500 units of antioxidant power.*

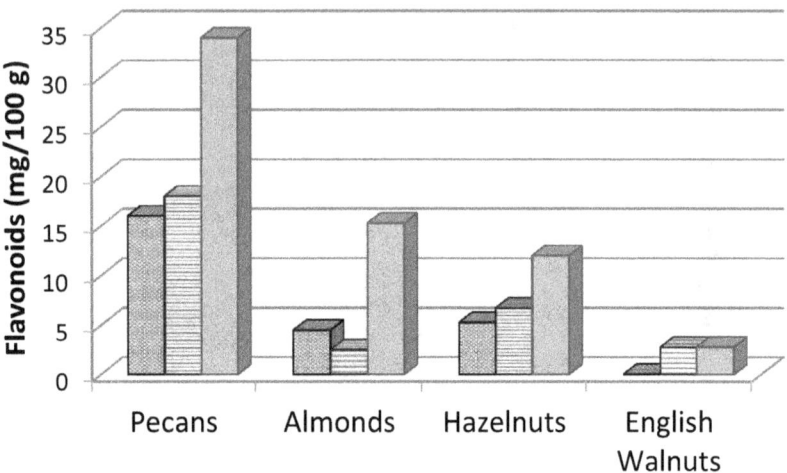

Figure 2.5. Pecans contain more flavonoids than other common nuts. Flavonoids are phenolic compounds that are also measured in the tests shown in Figures 2.3 and 2.4. From left to right, the three bars indicate flavan-3-ols, anthocyanins, and total flavanoids [7].

This antioxidant value puts pecans on an elite list of power foods that help the body defend against oxygen radicals, as suggested in **Figure 2.6**. Needless to say, potato chips, French fries, hamburgers, and most carbonated beverages are on the <u>bottom</u> of the list of antioxidant foods.

Brief Definitions of Major Phytochemicals

Bioflavonoids or Flavonoids- Flavonoids belong to a very diverse group of phytochemicals that contain a flavone ring. These substances are polyphenolic compounds. There are thousands of them in the plant kingdom. Some examples found in pecans are shown in **Figure 2.7**.

Phenolics- The total phenolic content of a plant product is used as a standardized laboratory measure because it provides a single total value for very complex mixtures of phytophenolics, all containing one or more phenolic rings.

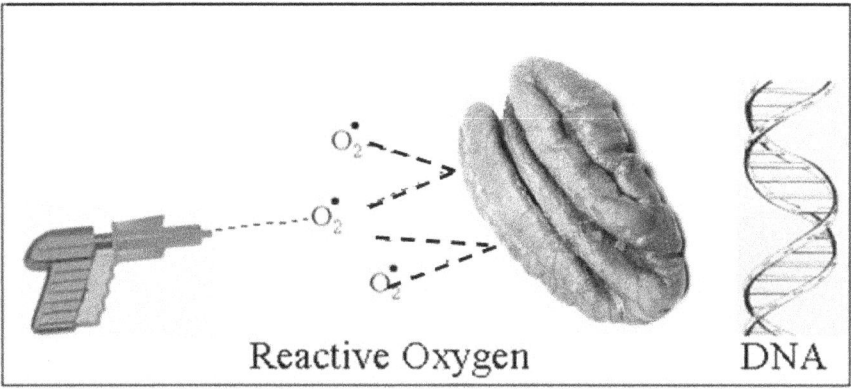

Figure 2.6. Daily metabolism generates a large amount of free radicals, as depicted by the Radical Gun at left. Antioxidants in pecans block these dangerous compounds before they can damage DNA and other cell parts.

Polyphenolics is a term that refers to general structures of molecules that have two or more phenolic rings in the structure. Flavonoids and bioflavonoids are polyphenolic compounds. Most of the categories shown in Figure 2.1 are polyphenolics and will be measured in the estimation of total phenolics.

Catechins are monomeric flavanols (flavan-3-ols). Catechins and epicatechins exist in pecans. These are used as building blocks to form proanthocyanidins (also called condensed tannins). Several of these catechin units link together to form larger molecules called oligomeric proanthocyanidins (OPCs). Pecan kernels are a rich source of OPCs.

Anthocyanidins are the aglycones (no sugar molecule attached) of the corresponding anthocyanins. Examples of anthocyanidins are the purple, blue and pink pigments called cyanidin, delphinidin, peonidin, petunidin and malvidin.

Proanthocyanidin molecules are built up using catechin units to make dimers and trimers (2 and 3 units) that are linked together (**Figure 2.7**). These are abundant in pecan kernels, especially in the dark coating, where they provide that characteristic pecan astringency.

Oligomeric Proanthocyanidins (OPCs) are 3 or more proanthocyanidins linked together. These are abundant in pecan kernels.

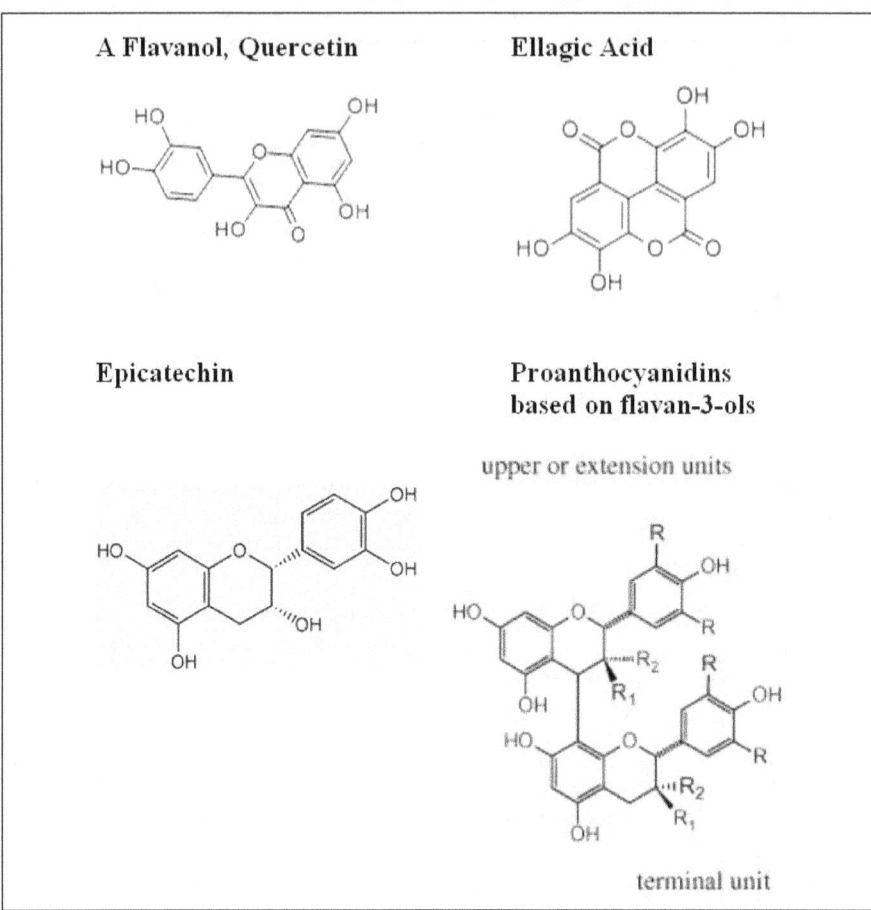

Figure 2.7. A few of the polyphenols found in pecans are shown in this figure.

Anthocyanins are anthocyanidins with a sugar molecule attached. Nature likes to attach sugar molecules to the anthocyanidins. Pecans contain largely cyanidin 3-O-glycosides.

Stilbenes are plant defense molecules called alexins. The stilbene compounds are synthesized by the plant for defense against pathogens, UV radiation, and other stresses. One of the best known stilbenes is resveratrol. Pecans and other tree nuts do not contain much resveratrol. Red wine is one of the best sources. Peanuts (ground nuts) have the highest level among nuts. The best source of resveratrol used in food supplements is the root of the Japanese knotweed called *Polygonum cuspidatum.*

Health Benefits of Flavonoids- In general, flavonoids are good antioxidants. The plants that make them use them not only for antioxidant protection, but also for protection against damage from ultraviolet radiation, environmental stresses, fungi and bacteria. As antioxidants, these substances can directly quench oxidative free radicals. Flavonoids can chelate (bind) metal ions that are often the catalysts for production of free radicals. Once chelated, the free metal ion becomes inactive. Chelation mechanisms can decrease the oxidative stress of free iron and copper ions.

Beyond Antioxidant Actions- Flavonoids have more profound effects within the human body than can be explained by simple antioxidant or chelation activity. It is now known that these plant substances help cells to regulate gene expression in very beneficial ways, and every major health agency recommends a high daily intake of the nuts, whole grains, fruits and vegetables that contain the diverse phytochemicals discussed in this chapter.

One way to look at chronic disease states like atherosclerosis, cancer, diabetes, or inflammatory and degenerative diseases is that they involve chronically adverse patterns of gene expression. As biologists have studied complex pathways involved in controlling the signals for regulating gene expression, it has become more and more obvious that phytochemicals in the diet play a major role in modulating these control systems. Flavonoids are not nutrients, not vitamins, not building blocks like essential amino acids or fatty acids. Yet, these so-called non-nutrients are powerful regulators of healthy gene expression patterns. Some of the pathways that can be modulated by flavonoids can control growth, proliferation and death of cancer cells.

Disease Prevention by Flavonoids- Patterns are emerging from major epidemiological studies that diets highly enriched with flavonoids are protective against coronary heart disease, atherosclerosis in major arteries, cancer, neurodegenerative diseases and inflammatory diseases in general. Pecans make an excellent contribution to a disease prevention diet strategy.

Take Home Messages The last USDA Food Guide Pyramid made recommendations for eating highly colored and flavorful fruits, vegetables, whole grains, nuts and legumes. Unfortunately, the guide was very hard to use and it was abandoned for the much simpler MyPlate concept.

Even though the US Dietary Guidelines still emphasize the need to eat more whole foods from all the categories shown in Figure 2.2, MyPlate does not do justice to antioxidant power foods including nuts, berries, dark green leafy vegetables and cereal brans. The Dietary Approach to Stop Hypertension does a better job, but does not depict advice in a pictorial way.

Every time you snack on pecans and other nuts instead of chips or cookies, you are making a power choice. To benefit from the full range of plant antioxidants, it is important to include berries, whole grain cereals, and an occasional dark chocolate bar. A true Power Bar may include all these ingredients. Pecans fit with other nutritional power foods for breakfast, lunch, snacks, supper and desserts.

Chapter 3

Pecans Improve Heart & Blood Vessel Health

Nuts Improve Heart Health- Pecans and other nuts protect the heart and cardiovascular system and decrease the risk of fatal heart disease. The lowered risk translates to an increased lifespan of about 2 years for people who regularly consume five or more servings of nuts per week. That single fact should convince most people to eat nuts regularly. However, researchers are interested in knowing why nuts improve heart health, and whether there are specific nutrients that produce the most benefit.

Figure 3.1 summarizes risk reduction due to nut consumption in large epidemiological investigations that include the Nurses' Health Study and the Health Professionals Follow-Up [14, 15]. Studies of diet and disease assign a general risk of 1.0 for the whole population.

High risk is defined as being significantly greater than 1, and reduced risk is less than 1.0. However, a generic Western diet pattern *increased the relative risk for heart disease* to 1.64. Processed meat consumption was one factor in this elevated risk, and all red meat had an average risk. Other dietary factors that increase risk are higher consumption of sugar, refined grain products, table salt and soft drinks.

However, regular consumption of nuts *lowered risk* significantly to a level of about 0.62. The reduced risk of heart disease due to regular nut consumption is independent of benefits obtained from consuming whole grains, fruits and vegetables. Take home message? A prudent diet includes regular consumption of nuts, whole grains, legumes, fruits, vegetables and fresh fish.

This chapter will explore the many reasons that pecans and other nuts improve heart health.

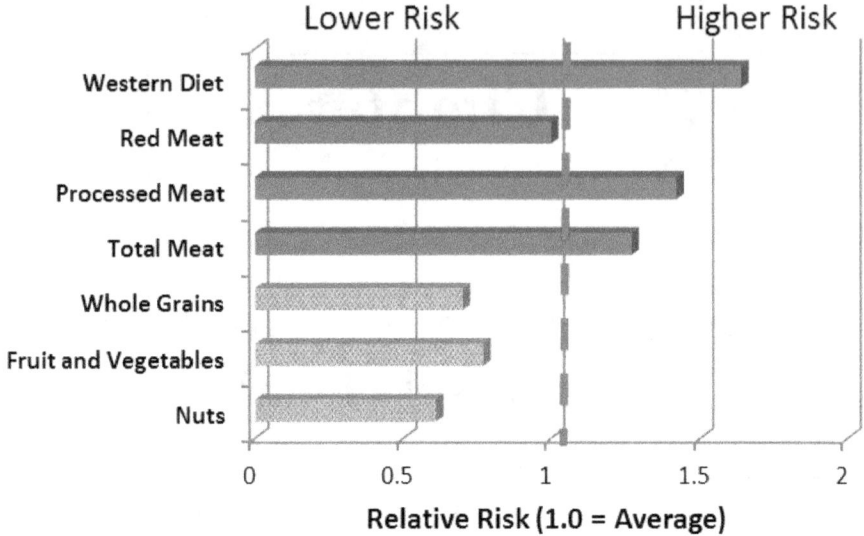

Figure 3.1. Nut consumption decreases risk for heart disease compared to a Western diet pattern that includes foods with saturated fat, trans fat, sugar, sodium, refined flour and processed meats. The effect of nut consumption (five or more servings per week) is independent of other dietary variables. Vertical line indicates average risk of 1.0.

The Healthy Fat Hypothesis Good heart health comes from a number of factors, including healthy coronary arteries, normal blood pressure, low tendency for blood to clot, and healthy cholesterol levels. Pecans contain several nutrients and phytochemicals that affect total heart health. However, the fact that nuts contain high levels of unsaturated fats and very low levels of saturated fats is almost certainly one element that reduces risk.

Saturated fats (SFA) are solid at room temperature. SFA include fats in butter, lard, and meats, as well as *trans* fats made by chemical treatment of vegetable oils. Some SFA are considered unhealthy because people who consume higher amounts tend to have higher cholesterol in the bloodstream. Monounsaturated fats (MUFA) have one double bond and are liquid at room temperature. MUFA do not raise cholesterol. Two rich sources of MUFA are olive oil and avocados. Polyunsaturated fats (PUFA) are oils that are also liquid at room temperature. PUFA lower cholesterol in the bloodstream and are considered heart healthy at normal levels of intake (1-2 tablespoons per day). PUFA are abundant in salad oils, cooking oils, whole grains, nuts and seeds.

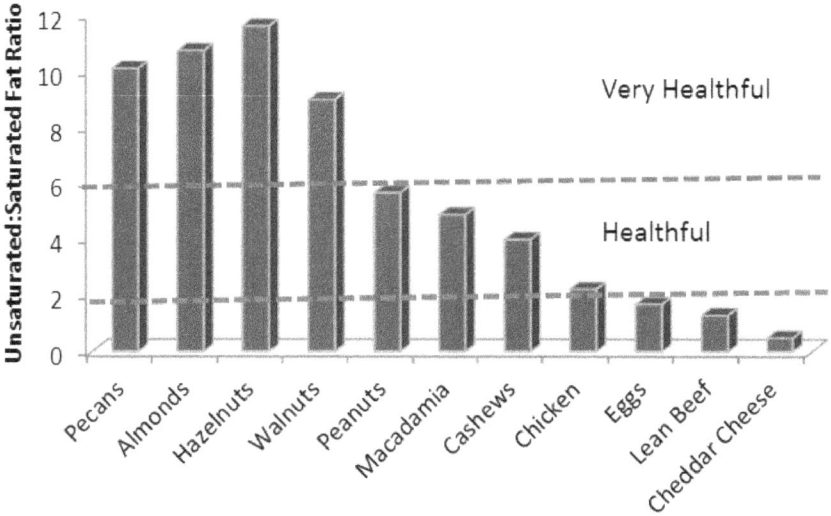

Figure 3.2. The reason that pecans and most other nuts help maintain healthy cholesterol is that they have ten times more *unsaturated fats* than saturated fats. Unsaturated fats tend to lower cholesterol, whereas the higher saturated fat level in beef and cheddar cheese tends to increase cholesterol. Values based on report of Sabate' and Wien (2010).

The very high level of unsaturated fats (UFA, the sum of MUFA plus PUFA) relative to saturated fats in pecans, almonds, hazelnuts and walnuts is shown in **Figure 3.2.** In these nuts, there is 10 times more UFA than SFA! The UFA:SFA in chicken and eggs is about 2, which is regarded as healthful but not as protective as nuts. However, animal meats, cheeses and other dairy products have more SFA than UFA. These levels are not protective for heart health in comparison to levels in pecans and other nuts.

Most researchers think that eating nuts five times a week improves heart health because nuts lower total cholesterol in the blood, and also reduce blood pressure. The principle reason for the lowering of cholesterol is the excellent ratio of UFA:SFA, which increases the body's ability to eliminate cholesterol.

Crunchiness Makes Fats Good! If having a high unsaturated fat content was the only thing that made nuts healthy, a person could get the same benefit by swallowing cooking oil—a bad idea! Cooking oils have already been extracted from the seeds where nature made them. They are not whole foods.

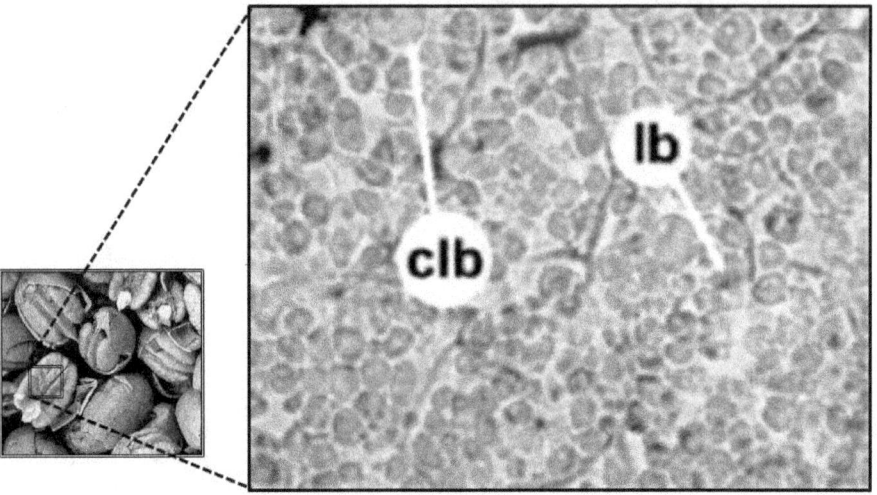

Figure 3.3. Lipids are stored within nut cells as tiny lipid bodies (lb) and central lipid bodies (clb)[16] in the microscopic view at right. Pecan lipids are inside of a crunchy food matrix that is completely unlike salad oils or cooking oils, which are liquids that lack matrix structure.

It is true that the fats in nuts are actually oils, and are liquid at room temperature. Pecan oil, almond oil, and peanut oil are sold in many stores. However, when growing nuts begin making oils, the oils are stored inside of cells in minute lipid droplets called "oil bodies". **Figure 3.3** shows a microscopic view of these oil bodies. The key point is that these tiny droplets are inside of nut tissues that provide the pleasant crunchy sensation when we eat nuts.

In past years, nuts were not recommended for good heart health because it was feared that the high fat content was a bad thing. This view has changed, and nuts are now on the "recommended" list for heart health. One reason for this is that fats found in whole nuts are not as absorbable as fats in cooking oils or in animal fats. A second reason is that fats in whole nuts improve the satisfying effect of a meal so a person tends to eat less food. Satiety is better when you eat pecans. As you can imagine, slurping cooking oil would not be enjoyable!

Omega-3 Essential Fatty Acids- Strong evidence supports the suggestion that omega-3 (also called n-3) fatty acids are required for total health, including heart health. Pecans contain a small amount of n-3 fatty acids, but the only natural nut with enough to improve heart health is probably the walnut.

However, the n-3 fatty acid in walnuts is a shorter version of the long-chain n-3 fatty acids in fish, where the evidence for heart health is clearest.

Pecans can readily be combined with high n-3 whole foods, especially fish. Pecan encrusted baked fish comes to mind, which combines healthy qualities of pecans with naturally high n-3 fatty acids in fish. There is nothing more powerful for health than combining several power foods in one meal!

Pecans, Cholesterol and Blood Lipids- Most medical doctors and scientists want to know how a treatment benefits heart health. Elevated cholesterol and triglycerides (TG) are well established markers for heart disease. One of the main ideas about the health benefits of pecans and other nuts is that they improve heart health partly because they lower total cholesterol, LDL-cholesterol, and TG. Also, LDL-cholesterol becomes "bad cholesterol" when it becomes oxidized, and there is evidence that pecan antioxidants prevent this process.

Medical research consistently shows that pecans lower total cholesterol, LDL-cholesterol, and TG in adults who have normal levels of these blood lipids. The first study to show this compared people who ate no nuts with a group that consumed 68 g of pecans a day (about two ounces) for an 8 week period [17]. LDL-cholesterol increased in the group eating no nuts but decreased in the group eating pecans. By the end of the study, LDL-cholesterol was 23% lower in the pecan group then in the controls.

Scientists at Loma Linda University evaluated the effect of pecan consumption on cholesterol in people following a Step 1 cholesterol-lowering diet that had been proposed by an expert panel of the National Cholesterol Education Program. The Step 1 diet is based on consumption of 30% of calories from fat. It is a relatively low fat, high carbohydrate approach that has the drawback of lowering "good" HDL-cholesterol and increasing "bad" TG. Subjects who consumed 72 g of pecans per day were eating more fat and less carbohydrate than the Step 1 diet—a good example of benefits of healthful fats!

The main result of the Loma Linda study was that a pecan-enriched diet significantly lowered total cholesterol, LDL-cholesterol and TG while increasing HDL-cholesterol. These changes are all consistent with better heart health. Strikingly, the lipid profile was improved even compared to the Step 1 diet that is intended to improve heart health! Adding pecans improved blood lipids even though total fat intake increased. Despite the increase in fat intake, subjects eating pecans did not gain significant body weight.

The observed health benefits of eating pecans cannot be explained just by the fact that pecans contain no cholesterol and have an excellent balance of unsaturated fats. Most researchers believe that the high levels of dietary fiber, magnesium, antioxidants and several phytochemicals all improve health.

Do Nuts Benefit People with High Cholesterol? The study that showed that nut consumption can add about 2 years to life expectancy in healthy people suggested that a greater benefit might be seen in people who already had chronic heart conditions or were overweight [1]. More research needs to be done to answer this important question.

Most studies on nut consumption, as well as studies on plant-based diets, suggest that nuts do improve the lipid profile in patients with high blood cholesterol [18, 19]. In addition, good heart health depends upon the health of the coronary arteries, which maintain blood flow to the actively beating heart tissues. It is paramount to prevent inflammation in the coronary blood vessels, prevent the build-up of plaque, and prevent blood from clotting in the major arteries of the heart. Let us examine how nut consumption affects some of these critical factors.

Pecans Block LDL Cholesterol Oxidation- LDL-cholesterol is not "bad" until it becomes oxidized to form ox-LDL or becomes modified in other ways. Pecans are a rich source of fat-soluble antioxidants that prevent this oxidation of LDL-cholesterol. In fact, pecans have tocopherols (relatives of vitamin E) that are carried in the LDL lipoprotein particle. These antioxidants are present exactly where they are needed to block the production of ox-LDL cholesterol. Let us look at why this is a health benefit of eating pecans.

Ox-LDL is toxic to cells that line blood vessels. In addition, ox-LDL enters the tissues underneath the blood vessel lining. In this space, immune cells called macrophages are programmed to ingest bacteria, cellular debris and LDL particles in the walls of blood vessels. In fact, they seem to prefer ox-LDL particles[20]. When macrophages ingest enough ox-LDL, they die in place and deposit their load of **cholesterol** to help build up atherosclerotic plaques.

When plaque grows, its components can be exposed directly to the blood and activate blood clotting. Diets that include pecans, other nuts, berries, and whole grains help slow this down and maintain healthy blood vessel walls [21, 22]. Healthy vessels have less plaque, maintain normal blood pressure, and have less tendency to form clots. These factors reduce risk for heart disease and add more healthy years to life.

Pecans Help Improve Blood Flow-   Healthy blood vessels produce relaxing chemicals that prevent the blood vessel from constricting. When vessels are open, more blood flows to the tissues and tissues stay healthy.

One of the relaxing chemicals is called nitric oxide, and it is made from an amino acid (arginine) that is abundant in pecan protein. In general, plant proteins have abundant arginine, and production of nitric oxide from these foods may be a factor in heart health [23, 24]. Why not be direct and just say it? By keeping the heart healthy, pecan protein is good for your love life! In fact, it is good for health of all your tissues, because poor blood flow is a sign of poor health in the entire body.

Relax Blood Vessels to Keep Blood Pressure Normal- The health of endothelial cells that line the blood vessels is also important for keeping blood pressure normal. These lining cells of the blood vessel manufacture substances that relax the smooth muscle in the wall of the artery. As arteries are relaxed throughout the body, blood pressure decreases.

To maintain normal blood pressure, it is important to consider pecans as part of a total plan that is rich in taste and phytochemical content. Studies that led to the DASH meal plan showed that key elements were low sodium, high fiber, good levels of magnesium, low cholesterol, and high antioxidants [25]. Pecans fit the bill perfectly, but are best consumed in a diet that also includes whole grains, leafy green vegetables, fish, several servings of legumes a week, and highly colored fruits and vegetables.

Protect Against Inappropriate Blood Clotting- Damage to the endothelial cells that line blood vessels sets the stage for blood clotting. Healthy endothelial cells manufacture substances that inhibit platelet activation, thereby inhibiting local blood clotting. Since this clotting mechanism is what precipitates most heart attacks in atherosclerotic coronary vessels, the role of phytochemicals in protecting normal endothelial cell function is crucial to protect the heart.

If endothelial cells are damaged, less of the relaxing substances are produced. In addition, platelets are exposed to collagen fibrils in the underlying layer of the blood vessels. Collagen causes platelet aggregation and initiates clotting.

Preventing Inflammation Helps Prevent Atherosclerosis- Atherosclerosis is known to be an inflammatory disease, which means that the immune system attempts to repair microscopic damage to the blood vessel walls. Even though

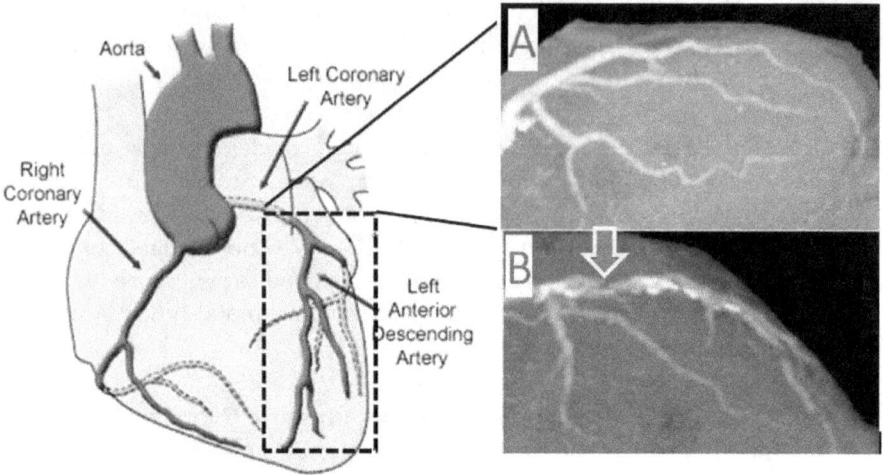

Figure 3.4. Regular nut consumption slows atherosclerosis and hardening of the coronary arteries. A major source of heart attacks is the "widow maker," the major artery supplying blood to the left side of the heart (in dashed rectangle at left). Panel A shows a healthy coronary artery with normal blood flow. Compare the healthy artery with the calcified blood vessel in panel B with blockage at the arrow. Figure based on images from the National Library of Medicine.

this is initially a healing process, it can get out of hand and actually create damage instead of repairing the tissues.

Damaged artery walls accumulate fatty deposits filled with lipid and oxidized LDL-cholesterol. What is worse, dying cells release calcium that mineralizes the fatty deposits. **Figure 3.4** compares a normal, healthy coronary artery in Panel A with one that is blocked and calcified (arrow in Panel B). This mineral is the reason that atherosclerosis literally means "hardening of the arteries." The tangle of lipid, calcium, and collagen fibrils activates blood clotting and greatly increases the likelihood that a blood clot will trigger a heart attack. It is encouraging that eating pecans and other smart choices can slow this process and help prevent the need to call an ambulance.

Nutrients and phytochemicals in nuts, other plant foods, and fish protect against inflammation in a myriad of ways. Antioxidants block oxidative stress that damages blood vessels and triggers inflammation. Omega-3 fatty acids reduce blood clotting by blocking platelet activation. Arginine is converted to nitric oxide to relax blood vessels and keep blood flowing to tissues.

Magnesium helps relax blood vessels and keeps blood pressure normal. Dietary fiber helps eliminate cholesterol from the body.

Pecans, Diet Quality and Total Heart Health- Whole foods have a nutritional balance that cannot be duplicated with prepared foods, refined foods, or food supplements. Pecans and other nuts provide important health benefits when they are substituted in the diet for poorer quality items such as salty or sugary snacks. In most diet studies, fats are exchanged for carbohydrates to maintain energy balance. When this is done, foods with unsaturated fats improve heart health whereas trans fats increase risk [26]. However, no single food item is a "miracle cure", and it is important to combine a variety of foods to create a healthy diet.

A simple example relative to heart health is that regular nut consumption creates a heart-healthy lipid profile, and this is particularly true when the nuts are substituted for snacks that contain high carbohydrate or trans fats. Nuts also tend to lower blood pressure and even improve cardiac output. However, an even greater total health benefit is possible. Grapes, berries, and pomegranates are all low fat foods with a high content of simple flavonoids. By combining nuts and berries in a balanced diet, blood lipid profile, blood pressure, and blood flow and blood vessel health are all improved [27, 28].

Pecans are "An Ounce of Prevention"- When consumed 2-5 times a week, pecans and other nuts contribute to heart health by improving blood lipid profiles, reducing oxidation of LDL-cholesterol, maintaining blood pressure, and fighting atherosclerosis. Pecans should be part of a "portfolio" for heart health that includes berries, leafy green vegetables, whole grains, and fresh fish for optimal heart health, for prevention of inflammation, and for better healing as we age or when tissue damage occurs for any reason. Evidence suggests that total health is improved the most by eating nuts and other plant-based foods, keeping body weight normal, and getting moderate exercise [1].

Web Resources

National Pecan Shellers Association Entrees,
http://www.ilovepecans.org/recipes_entrees.htm

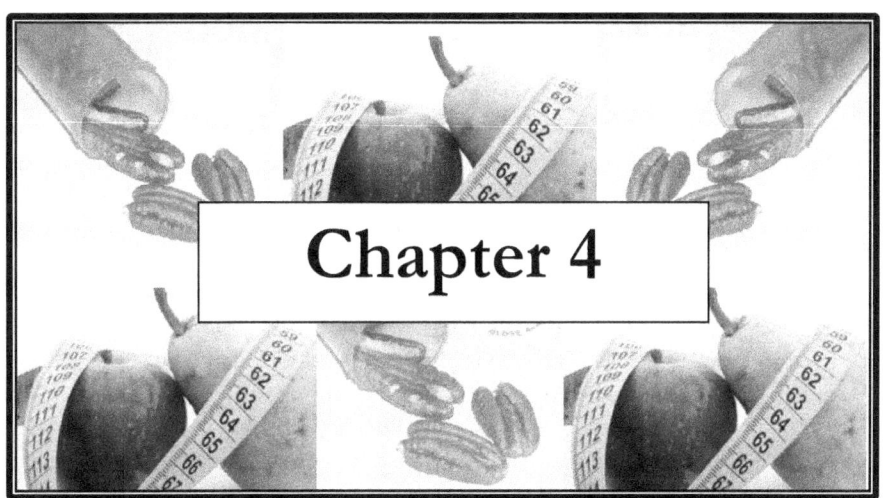

Chapter 4

Health Benefits of Pecans for Weight Control, Metabolic Syndrome, and Pre-Diabetes

Pecans Help Maintain Normal Body Weight- A surprising fact was discovered in several large studies that relate diet to health: People who consume the most nuts have the most optimal body weights, when compared to people who eat fewer nuts. They also tend to live the longest and are less affected by heart disease, high blood pressure and diabetes.

These studies did not ask what kinds of nuts were consumed, and there is no evidence that one kind is better than another. The major nuts consumed in the United States are almonds, walnuts, pecans, pistachios and peanuts (which is a legume but is counted as a nut owing to its nutrient composition).

Finding that nuts improve health and help maintain body weight seems a bit odd because all nuts are relatively high in fat, but it is easy to explain: Eating an ounce of nuts a few times a week adds healthy fats and improves the quality of the diet. It is the total diet that matters, and eating nuts need not increase fat or energy intake at all. As Dr. Walter Willett commented concerning dietary fat and heart disease [29]:

> "...total fat as a percent of energy is unimportant."

Pecans are High Fiber, Low Glycemic Foods- Pecans are an ideal food for weight maintenance. When eaten as part of a meal, the high content of dietary fiber and healthful fats slows stomach emptying and may decrease the secretion of a hunger hormone called ghrelin [30]. Because pecans have low carbohydrate content (especially the low simple sugar content), they keep blood glucose normal. When blood glucose is in the normal range, there is less secretion of insulin, a fat storing hormone. Therefore, there is less tendency to store energy from meals as fat.

The original concept of how individual foods affect blood glucose was called the glycemic index [31-33]. The change in blood glucose was measured after feeding an amount of food with a specific amount of carbohydrate. This was compared with the effect of 50 g of glucose, which was defined as 100. On this scale, pecans and other nuts have a very low glycemic index ranging from about 13-55 [32, 33].

A newer approach called "glycemic load" evaluates how much blood glucose rises after a defined meal, as calculated from the total carbohydrate and average glycemic index of foods in the meal [34, 35]. Nuts have very little effect on raising blood glucose and actually *lower* the glycemic load of carbohydrates in the same meals [36]. From a practical standpoint, it makes sense to use pecans as ingredients in salads, entrees and desserts because their ability to lower the glycemic load may lead to weight loss.

Pecans for Weight Reduction- When pecans are consumed as part of a diet designed to lower cholesterol, they do not produce weight gain [37, 38]. One study compared weight reduction caused by a low calorie diet (one that contains just over 1000 kcal/day) with either 84 g of nuts or an equivalent amount of complex carbohydrate. Even though the two diets had the same number of calories, subjects consuming nuts lost significantly greater weight (43 pounds vs. 26.6 pounds) after 24 weeks. Much of the weight loss was abdominal fat, because waist circumference decreased by 17 cm in the nut group compared to 12 cm in the carbohydrate group.

The take-home messages based on current research are simple. Adding nuts to a normal diet does not produce weight gain in most people. Also, nuts can be a valuable part of diets designed for weight loss because they help improve the feeling of fullness, improve heart health, and may assist weight loss due to lower absorption of fats from meals.

Fats in Nuts are Less Absorbable than Fats in Other Foods- The increased weight loss seen in subjects consuming nuts compared to complex carbohydrates caused researchers to test why this might be the case. In most foods more than 95% of the energy in fats is absorbed. However, for nuts, up to 25% of the food energy is <u>not absorbable</u> [39, 40]. Also, when subjects consume a low calorie diet with nuts, some energy is apparently excreted in the urine as high caloric ketone bodies [41]. If confirmed in more studies, these effects could help provide dieters with an edge for better weight loss.

Food Guides and Diet Plans that Recommend Pecans and Other Nuts-
Average US nut consumption is about 0.5 servings per week, which needs to be increased for better health. Pecans fit into dietary plans for anyone who is not allergic to nuts. Here are a few thoughtful, **evidence-based food guides** that suggest eating more nuts.

> **Dietary Approaches to Stop Hypertension**- Plan on 4-5 servings of nuts per week with a serving defined as 1/3 cup or 1.5 ounces of whole nuts to help maintain normal blood pressure.

> **US Dietary Guidelines 2010**- US nut consumption should be increased to 4-5 ounces per week for adults who are not allergic to nuts. For a 2000 calorie diet, 4 ounces is recommended.

> **Mayo Clinic/Mediterranean Food Guide**- Based on the PREDIMED study, up to a handful of nuts per day should be included with legumes, fruits and vegetables at most meals to benefit heart health and prevent diabetes.

> **Harvard Healthy Eating Pyramid**- A variety of nuts, seeds, legumes, and soy (tofu) should be included in the daily diet as sources of healthy fats, plant protein, fiber, antioxidant phytochemicals and minerals. Substitute nuts for less nutritious snacks to keep calories in balance.

> **American Heart Association/Heart & Stroke Foundation "Go Nuts for Health"**- Eat 3 to 5 servings per week of nuts, seeds, and legumes. One serving is 1/3 cup of nuts, ½ cup of dry beans, or 2 tablespoons of peanut butter.

> **National Cancer Institute**- Include some meatless meals each week, using legumes, nuts and soy to enhance protein quality.

Dr. Weil's Anti-Inflammatory Diet Pyramid- Eat moderate amounts of nuts as sources for healthy fats and protein. Raw nuts are best. If toasted or chopped, use immediately to prevent rancidity.

University of Michigan Healing Foods Pyramid- Choose a variety of nuts as sources of healthful monounsaturated fats and other nutrients.

WebMD's "Ounce of Prevention"- Replace snack foods with 1 ounce of a variety of nuts, keeping in mind the fact that nuts contain about 160-200 calories per ounce.

The experts agree, pecans and other nuts fit any diet plan or cuisine that emphasizes healthful fats and low glycemic load. Do remember that one ounce of pecans contains 200 calories of food energy, so it is best to substitute nuts for other, less *nut*ritious foods such as potato chips and sodas that have higher glycemic responses.

What is the Metabolic Syndrome?- As children and adults in the US have become fatter, the incidence of metabolic syndrome has increased. Metabolic syndrome is characterized by impaired glucose tolerance, decreased insulin sensitivity, high blood glucose, and a high-risk blood lipid profile (lower HDL-cholesterol, high triglycerides and usually elevated LDL and total cholesterol). In addition abdominal obesity and hypertension are often present (see risk factors in Table 4.1).

Table 4.1. Indications of the Metabolic Syndrome (3 or more)

Waistline in women	> 35 inches
Waistline in men	> 40 inches
Blood pressure	> 135/85 mm Hg
Fasting blood glucose	> 110 mg/dl
HDL cholesterol-women	< 50 mg/dl
HDL cholesterol-men	< 40 mg/dl
Fasting triglycerides	> 150 mg/dl

Persons with metabolic syndrome have a marked risk of developing overt diabetes, heart disease, atherosclerosis and stroke. Metabolic syndrome has reached epidemic proportions in the U.S. and other countries that are wealthy enough to provide modern, calorific diets while maintaining relatively sedentary work and life styles. Europeans have decided to find a solution with the LIPGENE research project [42, 43]. **The goal is to develop a strategy to alter dietary patterns to prevent metabolic syndrome. European estimates suggest that 10-20% of current middle-aged and elderly men and 10-25% of middle-aged to elderly women have metabolic syndrome. US statistics are much higher, perhaps twice this rate. Fortunately, this epidemic is a *reversible* tragedy in our opinion.**

The movie, "Super-Size Me," depicts a man who put himself into severe metabolic syndrome in just 30 days by eating a fast food diet. Most Americans under the age or 50 have now been eating fast food and phytochemical-depleted processed foods all their lives. One point illustrated particularly well in "Super-Size Me" is that *it is easier to get into metabolic syndrome than to get out again.*

Pecans and Other Nuts Help Reverse Metabolic Syndrome- Can pecans and other nuts make a difference in reversing metabolic syndrome? Evidence shows that the answer is YES. Healthful fats, antioxidants, fiber and phytochemicals in nuts, legumes, fruit and vegetables can benefit health by improving fasting blood glucose, fasting triglycerides, blood pressure, and helping reduce body weight and the waistline. Nuts help normalize all of the criteria for Metabolic Syndrome except for raising HDL-cholesterol. Lack of an effect on HDL-cholesterol is offset by the ability to lower LDL-cholesterol and improve the ratio of "good" to "bad" cholesterol. Pecans and other nuts help fight metabolic syndrome in all these ways:

1. **Decreasing blood glucose**
2. **Decreasing insulin resistance**
3. **Protecting large blood vessels**
4. **Decreasing oxidative stress**
5. **Having anti-inflammatory actions**
6. **Decreasing the oxidizability and oxidation of LDL-cholesterol**
7. **Relaxing blood vessels and lowering blood pressure**

Pecans in a Dietary "Portfolio" to Fight Metabolic Syndrome- Including more pecans and other nuts in an eating plan for weight maintenance does improve several risk factors for Metabolic Syndrome. However, for people who are overweight, by far the greatest benefit arises from weight loss, and particularly loss of abdominal fat. Waistline control is critical. The definitions for waist circumference in Table 4.1 are for people in the US and Europe. Other groups, especially Asians, can be overweight at these levels.

Nuts "have a tendency to lower body weight and fat mass" according to researchers who have studied the association [38]. However, to make this a certainty, overweight people need to make sure they are eating fewer calories [41] or adding significant physical activity to their daily routines [44].

Surprisingly, a moderate-fat, diet containing nuts and peanut butter provided more weight loss and higher participation than a low-fat diet when women and men ate 1200 and 1500 calories per day, respectively [45]. Subjects who increased nut consumption by half a serving per day and increased peanut butter consumption by 0.7 servings per day lost 9 cm from their waistline over 18 months compared to 4.8 cm for the low-fat group that did not add nuts.

A moderate-fat vegetarian diet in which nuts provided the majority of fats decreased signs of the metabolic syndrome more than a high-carbohydrate vegetarian diet even though weight loss was not different. The diet with added nuts and soy products produced greater satiety, lower cholesterol, and lower triglycerides [18, 46]. In this study, the main marker of inflammation (hsCRP, high sensitivity C-Reactive Protein) decreased but was not different between groups (note that weight loss itself is anti-inflammatory). To obtain these benefits, energy intake was reduced to 60% of daily requirements, and diets were prepared by dietitians in a clinic along with professional weight loss counseling.

Pecans for Low Glycemic Snacks- Nuts not only have a very low glycemic index, they lower the glycemic load of foods with higher glycemic effects when eaten together. The greatest benefit of eating pecans comes when the nuts are substituted for less nutritious foods. For example, Figure 4.1 shows a snack of pecans and dried cranberries that have a low glycemic index. In contrast, a serving of potato chips with a beverage sweetened with high fructose corn sweetener has a much higher glycemic index and will evoke a rise in blood glucose and insulin. The lemon in the ice water is a reminder that acidic foods also delay stomach emptying and lower the glycemic response.

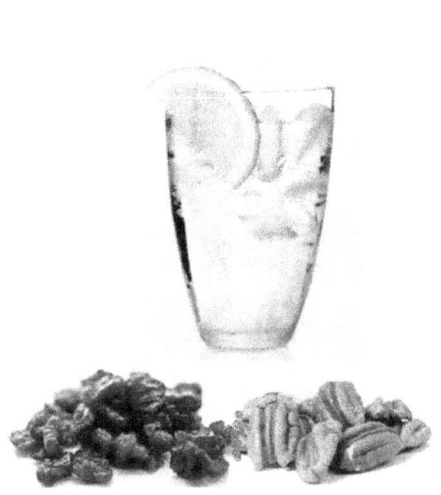 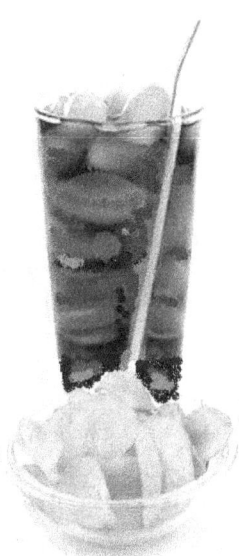

Figure 4.1. Examples of low glycemic versus high glycemic snacks. Pecans and cranberries with ice water help lose weight compared to potato chips and a soft drink that cause weight gain.

Other Phytochemicals Assist Blood Glucose Control- Pecans and other nuts provide a number of benefits but are complemented by the numerous simple flavonoids and carotenoids in berries, fruits and vegetables. Clifford [47] reviewed the literature on dietary phenols, polyphenols and tannins of the kind found in pecans. He concluded that one of the most promising benefits of these compounds would be in improving blood glucose control and treating symptoms of the Metabolic Syndrome.

Proanthocyanidins Delay Starch Digestion and Fight High Glucose- Having high proanthocyanidins (PACs) is one of several reasons that pecans delay the increase of blood glucose after a meal. The reason for this is that starch digestion requires an enzyme called amylase that PACs partially inactivate. In addition to pecans, several other foods contain PACs, but some of these, such as high-tannin sorghum grain, are not consumed in the US.

For people with high blood glucose, a drug called acarbose is sometimes prescribed to block starch digestion. People who eat pecans and other sources of PACs are getting natural starch blockers in their meals without taking drugs. The high content of PACs is one reason that pecans have more antioxidant power than walnuts (**Figure 2.3**). PACs are abundant in some whole foods and spices, but are absent from nearly all refined US foods [48, 49]. That is why the average US intake is very low, about 49-71 mg of PACs per day. Needless to say, a snack based on potato chips and a soft drink has zero PACs, unlike the high levels in a handful of pecans and cranberries.

Prevention of Type 2 Diabetes- There is no single dietary or lifestyle factor, including nuts, that can prevent Type 2 diabetes. However, Type 2 diabetes can be prevented or reversed when initially overweight or obese people combine a low calorie, plant based diet with adequate weekly exercise. In fact, a vigorous lifestyle intervention showed greater improvement in the Diabetes Prevention trial than a drug for diabetes treatment called metformin [44]. Based partly on this work, the consensus is that most Type 2 diabetes can be prevented if it is caught early enough, and reversed if it has already begun [44, 50, 51]. Preventing diabetes is important because long-term damage to the health of the kidneys, heart and eyes cannot be restored.

Nut consumption can assist with blood glucose control, weight loss and changes in cardiovascular system that are needed for prevention of adult-type diabetes. Because long-term consequences of diabetes are very serious (blindness, kidney failure, and stroke), successful interventions must be vigorous. A combined program with medical supervision by a physician and diabetes educator is needed for most people.

If diabetes mellitus continues, dealing with it either requires life-long drug treatment or gastric bypass surgery [52]. Frankly, a program that includes nuts, berries, and weight reduction seems much less drastic.

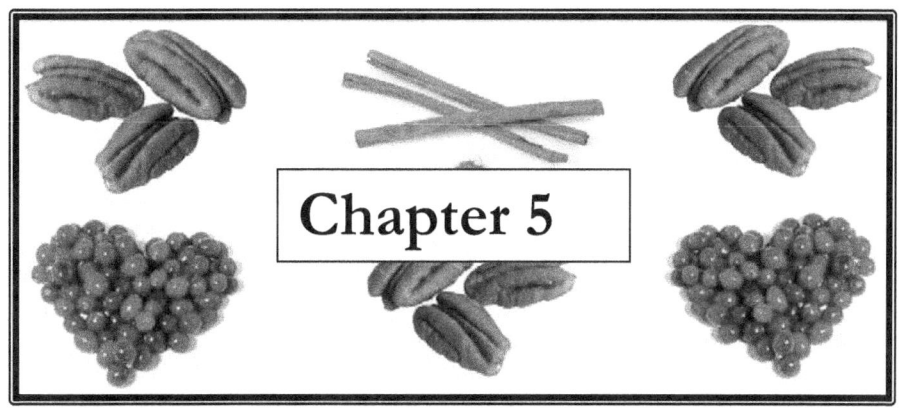

Chapter 5

Pecans "Phyte" Against
Inflammatory Diseases

Pecans are excellent choices that fit within a variety of anti-inflammatory diets and lifestyles (inflammation is not just about what we eat, it is how we adapt to stress and how we deal with trauma). This chapter will explain current thinking based on new studies of inflammation.

Healing and Fighting Inflammation are Two Sides of the Same Coin- It is no coincidence that "heal" is literally the root of "health." And healing always involves cells of the immune system moving into tissues to clean up cellular debris before other cells can make repairs. When this happens on a microscopic level, it is a very good thing. However, the immune system can overreact. When immune cells cause more blood to flow to part of the body, that is good. But immune signals also make blood vessels leaky, and tissues swell up around an injury. More blood flow makes the tissues warm, the skin turns red in around the injury, and released substances cause pain. Redness, swelling, heat and pain are classic outward signs of local inflammation, a tissue reaction involving the immune system.

We are all familiar with inflammation of the skin caused by cuts, stings and bites. *Fewer people know that the entire gastrointestinal tract is a major source of inflammation* that we can counteract with personal dietary choices, or make worse through uninformed choices.

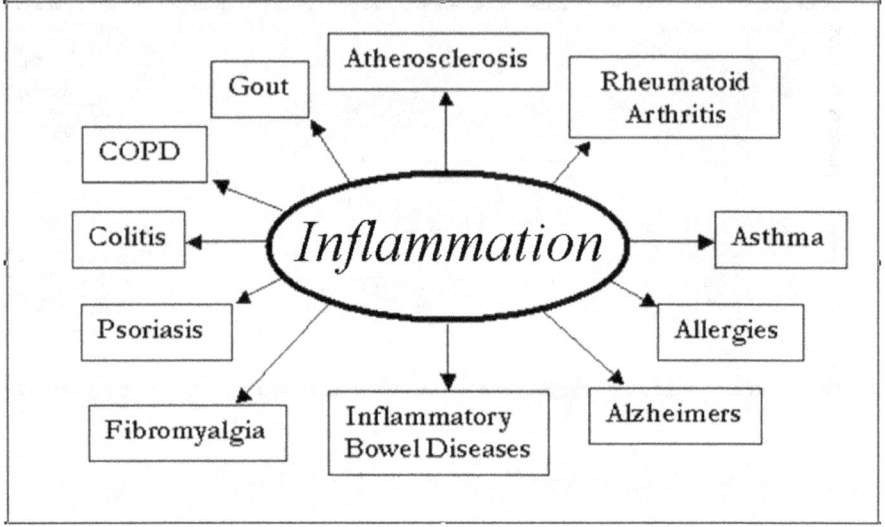

Figure 5.1. Anti-inflammatory actions of phytochemicals in pecans as part of a dietary portfolio suppress synthesis and release of cytokines that are major regulators in multiple chronic inflammatory diseases shown here.

Most major diseases involve inflammation and loss of function, and some examples are shown in **Figure 5.1**. Many inflammatory conditions have the suffix "itis" attached to their medical names, such as arthritis, gingivitis, prostatitis, dermatitis, bronchitis, enteritis, colitis, hepatitis, pancreatitis and asthma (the exception that proves the rule!) These conditions over-activate the immune system, which releases substances and signals that lead to aches and pains distant from the original inflammation.

The good news is that pecans are part of an anti-inflammatory diet that supports the microscopic, healing work of the immune system in the gastrointestinal tract and blood vessels, yet helps keep the system in balance and prevents loss of function.

Meals Can Promote Inflammation, but Nuts Protect Blood Vessels After Meals- As meals are digested and nutrients are absorbed, various inflammatory mediators increase in the blood stream and affect the health of blood vessels. The effect of single meals is not generally a problem, but over a lifetime, there can be damage to blood vessel walls. Healthful fats of the kinds found in nuts can reduce this inflammatory response [53]. In addition, nut consumption increases plasma antioxidant levels after meals [22]. Needless to say, protecting blood vessel health is a good thing for every part of the body.

Anti-Inflammatory Traditions- Diets that promote long life have been found to be anti-inflammatory, and the best known approaches for which there is evidence of increased longevity are the Okinawa approach and the Mediterranean plan (knowing that there are hundreds of ways to create a Mediterranean- or Japanese-style diet). However, you don't need to travel abroad to live a long, healthy life. The "California style" incorporated in the Adventist Health Study led to a greater average life expectancy than any of the international approaches. Men and women at lowest risk lived, on average, to 83 and 85 years, respectively. And one of the cornerstones of the advice remains, eat nuts 4-5 times a week.

Anti-Inflammatory Food Guides- Any dietary approach that promotes long life fights inflammation while preserving healthy immune function. In fact, in a hospital setting, loss of immune function is a very serious sign that prognosis is poor. Clinical nutritionists are very interested in dietary approaches to combat inflammation [54]. But even for healthy people, day-to-day choices reduce inflammation, promote normal tissue turnover, and preserve immune function.

Dr. Andrew Weil has explicitly developed an anti-inflammatory eating plan based on his medical knowledge [55]. Similarly, the University of Michigan has developed a *healing food pyramid*. And the evidence-based Harvard Nutrition Source recognizes immune support as a nutritional goal and makes recommendations based on scientific evidence [56]. Each of these food guides recognizes the importance of eating nuts several times a week, especially when the nuts replace chips, fries, sweets or animal fats.

Antioxidant and Anti-Inflammatory Power are Two Different Things- Any nutrient that can bind an unpaired electron or free radical is an antioxidant, but that does not mean it fights inflammation. Among pecan phytochemicals, the ones with the highest anti-inflammatory power are the fat soluble relatives of vitamin E, the flavonoids such as quercetin, and the proanthocyanidins that you taste when you bite into pecan kernels.

An anti-inflammatory diet should contain several high PAC foods on a daily basis. Cacao beans are a rich source, and dark chocolate in moderation adds PACs. In addition to the foods shown in **Figure 5.2**, cinnamon is a very rich source, providing about 81 mg of PAC per gram.

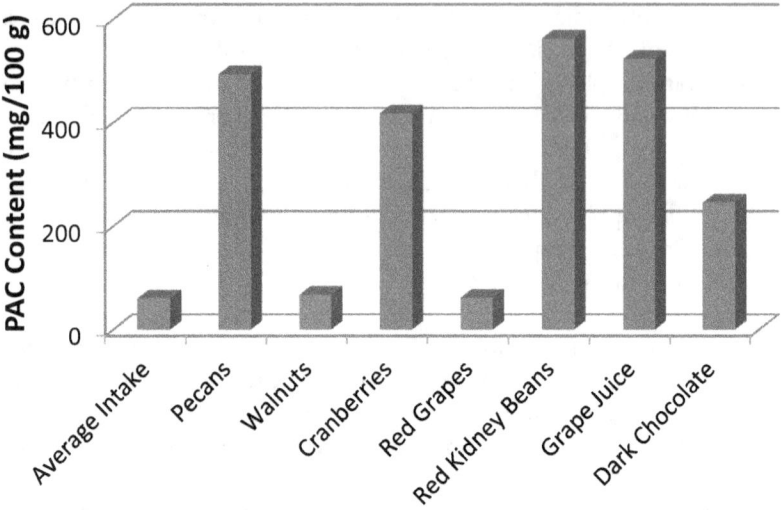

Figure 5.2. Proanthocyanidins in foods and in the US diet. The foods shown are all high in PACs compared to most other US foods, because average intake of PACs among US adults ranges from 49-71 mg/day. *One serving of pecans would more than double the intake.* Other good sources are cranberries, kidney beans, grape juice and dark chocolate.

The effect of cinnamon on blood sugar was discovered when Dr. Robert Anderson noticed that apple pie did not raise blood glucose as much as expected. He tested apples to see if they blocked the rise in blood glucose (due to the sugar in the pies). When that did not work, he tested cinnamon and found that the effect was due to a PAC [57]. Putting 1 gram of cinnamon (half a teaspoon) on yogurt or breakfast cereal is a good health practice.

PACs are found in short and long forms in two types called A and B. The majority in pecans are longer chain length, and have 10 or more PAC subunits. Current evidence suggests that short and long forms and A and B types have different effects. It seems prudent to eat a variety of whole foods and use a variety of spices to get optimum effects—such as spiced pecans with cranberries!

Abdominal Fat Makes Inflammation Worse- Inflammation is caused by cells of the immune system acting on other tissues. Fat cells are part of this system and release many products that make many diseases worse. For example, immune cells communicate by sending out protein messengers called cytokines.

The word cytokine means "to stimulate a cell." Fat cells in the abdomen produce cytokines called tumor necrosis factor α and interleukins 6 and 8, which are classic cytokines that are also made by cells of the immune system. Remember the watchword is to keep your waistline under 35 inches if you are a woman, and under 40 inches if you are a man. Diet and exercise are the best tools in the fight against fat-induced inflammation. The good news is that a person doesn't have to lose all the weight to see significant improvements. Just getting on an appropriate diet and beginning to lose weight with diet and exercise cause marked improvements [58, 59].

Don't Let Sugars Cross-Link Your Proteins- If glucose is a natural sugar, why it is important to keep blood sugar low? One reason is that simple sugars like glucose ("blood sugar") and fructose react with proteins. The sugars both bind to certain nitrogen groups (amino groups) in proteins in the blood and blood vessel walls. At first the reaction is reversible and does no harm. However, the bond can become permanent and change the shape of the protein, damaging it and activating the immune system in some cases.

Irreversible bonds between sugars and damaged proteins are called AGE proteins. The abbreviation is an intentional pun that stands for Advanced Glycation End-products. One form of an AGE protein is Hemoglobin A1c, a form of hemoglobin that has reacted with glucose. Normal levels of HbA1c should be less than 5%, but they increase above 6% and more in people with diabetes.

HbA1c is measured in a routine medical test that indicates to doctors whether a diabetic patient has controlled blood sugar over the past 100 days. The test is a marker for the damage caused by high blood sugar to blood vessels and other organs such as the kidneys, heart, eyes and nerves. AGE protein formation is one reason that people with diabetes frequently develop atherosclerosis and heart disease. Even with insulin treatment, life expectancy is cut short by about 15 years.

Proanthocyanidins in pecans and bioflavonoids in fruit and berries can help block the formation of AGE proteins, as shown in the laboratory test displayed in **Figure 5.3**. This is why daily consumption of nuts, fruits and berries is helpful as one part of a strategy for prevention and management of Type 2 diabetes mellitus. For someone who already has metabolic syndrome or diabetes, the total plan must be developed along with medical doctors and a health care team.

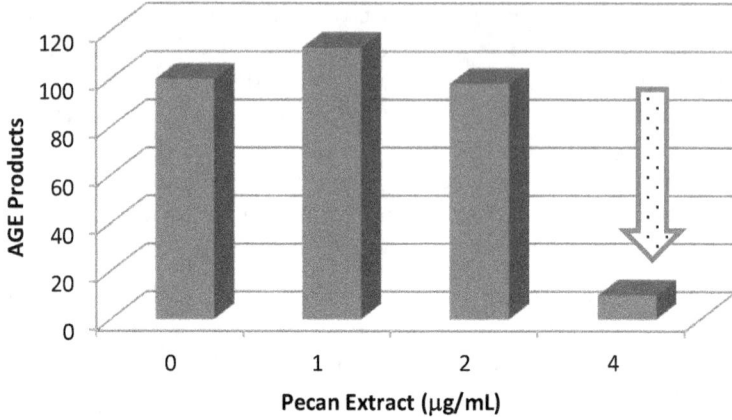

Figure 5.3. Pecan extract blocks the ability of fructose to glycate proteins in a laboratory test (indicated by arrow). Test results are courtesy of Dr. Phillip Greenspan.

The Inflammasome, How the Immune System Activates Inflammation-
With every meal we eat, the gastrointestinal tract is exposed to foreign substances and bacteria that must be detoxified and sterilized. The process begins in the stomach with its acid and anti-bacterial digestive enzymes. It continues in the small intestine with enzymes from the pancreas and bile from the liver. The immune system is poised to respond to potential pathogens, and more than half of the cells of the immune system are located in the tissues lining the stomach, small intestine and colon.

Recent scientific reports have shown that cells of the immune system recognize patterns that are either associated with pathogens (bacteria, viruses, and parasites), tissue damage, or foreign antigens. The system detects threats using a scaffold inside of immune cells called the inflammasome (**Figure 5.4**). When activated, the system secretes cytokines such as IL1-β (IL1-β), and recruits more immune cells. Fortunately, the inflammasome system has several elements that can be employed to improve personal health.

Firstly, saturated fats and glucose increase the sensitivity of the system. A larger immune response that is harder to control is not desirable, so diets comprised of whole foods like pecans that emphasize unsaturated fats and have little refined starch or sugars are good choices. Secondly, cholesterol crystals are one of the inflammasome activators, so it is useful that nuts and Mediterranean style

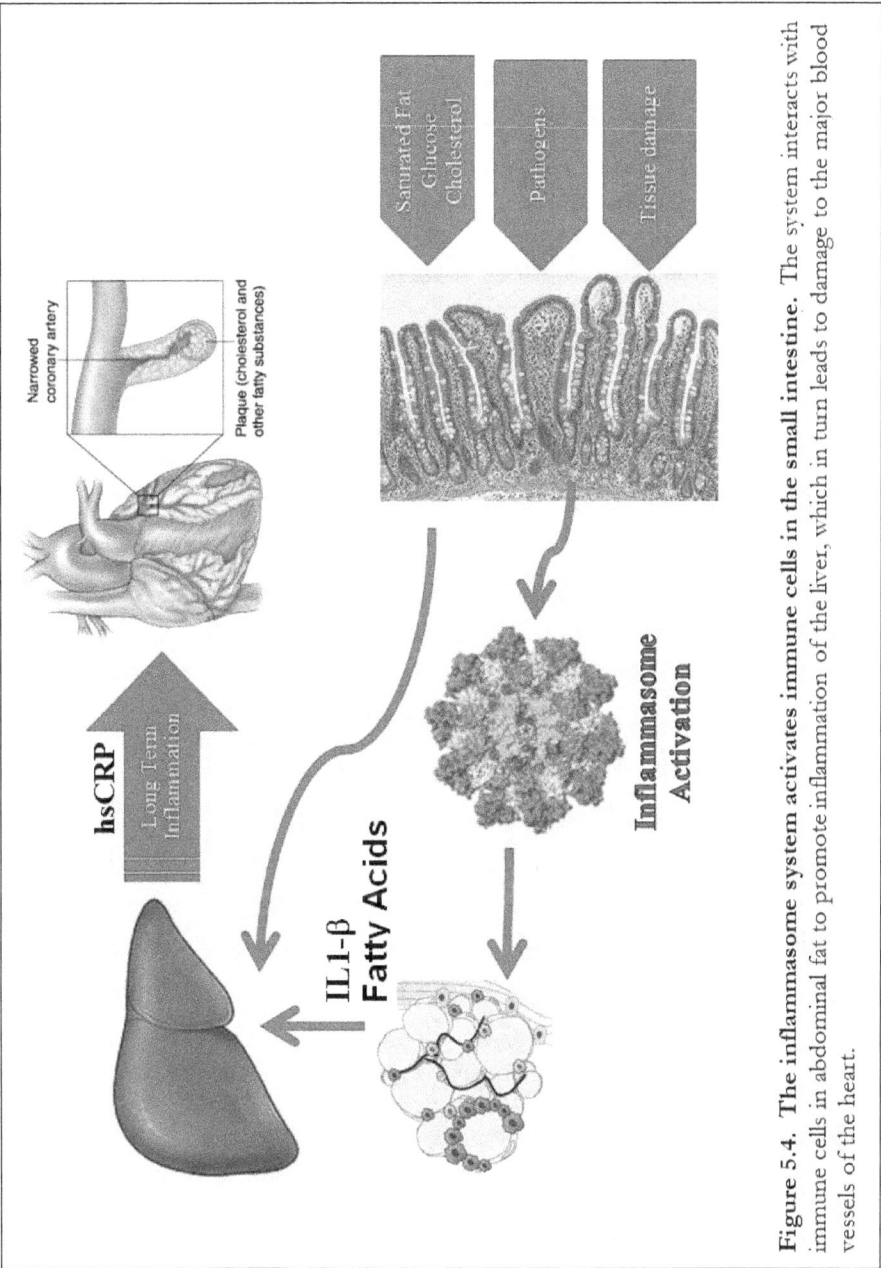

Figure 5.4. The inflammasome system activates immune cells in the small intestine. The system interacts with immune cells in abdominal fat to promote inflammation of the liver, which in turn leads to damage to the major blood vessels of the heart.

diets can lower cholesterol. Thirdly, antioxidant phytochemicals in pecans, berries, teas, and other foods keep a limit on how active the immune system can be, basically helping prevent over-reaction that leads to damage.

Clinical Markers for Systemic Inflammation- Figure 5.4 shows two markers of system-wide inflammation. Interleukin 1-β comes from immune cells in the small intestine and fat cells. C-reactive protein (CRP) is released from the liver and also from immune cells in inflammed blood vessels. CRP is now measured in blood tests to determine risk for cardiovascular disease. That is why most people with chronic inflammatory disease end up dying of heart attacks and strokes. Did you know that CRP is a much better predictor for who will have a heart attack than is LDL-cholesterol? A major problem in heart disease may be systemic inflammation [60-62]. Two reasons that aspirin is recommended for people with atherosclerotic disease is that it is anti-inflammatory and anti-platelet (decreases blood clotting). The trick with atherosclerotic disease is to cool down blood vessel inflammation, to keep plaques from destabilizing and also to keep blood clots from forming.

Pecan Phytochemicals Block NF-Kappa B Activation That Controls Inflammation- Pecans contain many substances that can block the activation of nuclear factor kappa B (NF-kB) and thereby suppress gene expression for many inflammatory molecules or enzymes. Inhibition of NF-kB has been shown for caffeic acid, quercetin, resveratrol and its derivatives, ellagic acid and its derivatives and proanthocyanidins.

NF-kappa B Activation, Endothelial Cell Activation and Leukocyte Transmigration- NF-kB activation controls gene expression for cell adhesion molecules. Therefore, it is not surprising that most of the substances listed above are inhibitors of NF-kB activation and will suppress gene expression of cell adhesion molecules in blood vessels. In this manner, inhibitors of NF-kB activation can suppress migration of white blood cells from blood to tissue. Since this basic mechanism is involved in heart disease and metastatic cancer, it should be no surprise that pecan phytochemicals are good preventive medicine for multiple conditions.

Protecting the Stomach Lining- Proanthocyanidins have been shown to protect the stomach lining during extreme experimental stress in rats[63]. Researchers subjected rats to water-immersion restraint stress. This treatment produces stomach ulcers in rats. If the rats have been taking proanthocyanidins in their drinking water, ulcer erosions are inhibited in a dose-dependent manner. The mechanism involved important anti-ulcer activities.

Antioxidant phytochemicals can protect the stomach from oxidative free radical damage. They scavenge free radicals present in foods and preservatives. It has been suggested that the stomach is a bioreactor and these oxidative free radicals can be absorbed and significantly impact the whole body. The presence of antioxidant phytochemicals in the diet makes a significant difference on what happens within the stomach[64]. Researchers have shown that increases in free radical concentration of oils or fats in meat in simulated gastric fluid could be blocked by catechin and polyphenols. This certainly suggests that high flavonoid intake at meals is highly protective during the early digestive processes in the stomach. For a review of the many types of reactions taking place in the stomach that can produce free radicals see [65].

Protecting the Small Intestine- The same polyphenolics that the pecan uses to protect itself from bacterial, viral or fungal attacks have anti-bacterial, anti-fungal and anti-viral properties in humans. This may be particularly important in the gastrointestinal tract, which is exposed to them in high concentrations. 60-70% of the immune system is present in the walls of the gut, waiting to defend us from "outsiders". The low pH of the stomach kills a lot of microorganisms, but when food moves into the small and large intestines, the pH is more favorable to bacterial growth. Also, protozoa can affect the condition of the gut wall. Any organism capable of aggravating the immune system sentinels in the wall of the gut can set up a gut inflammation; pecan polyphenolics should diminish this response.

Colon Health- The high content of insoluble dietary fiber and non-starch polysaccharides, as well as anti-inflammatory nature of pecan phytochemicals [66] makes pecans an excellent choice for colon health. In addition, pecans contain a variety of mild phytoestrogens that are converted to compounds called enterolignans [67]. These pecan nutrients together with good sources of soluble fiber (cereals and fruit) and probiotics help maintain a healthy population of microbes.

In the colon, chronic inflammation activates the inflammasome and immune system in a way that can contribute to development of colorectal cancer. Some features of this control are very different from what happens in the small intestine, owing to the presence of a large population of microbes in the healthy colon. These differences will be discussed in the next chapter.

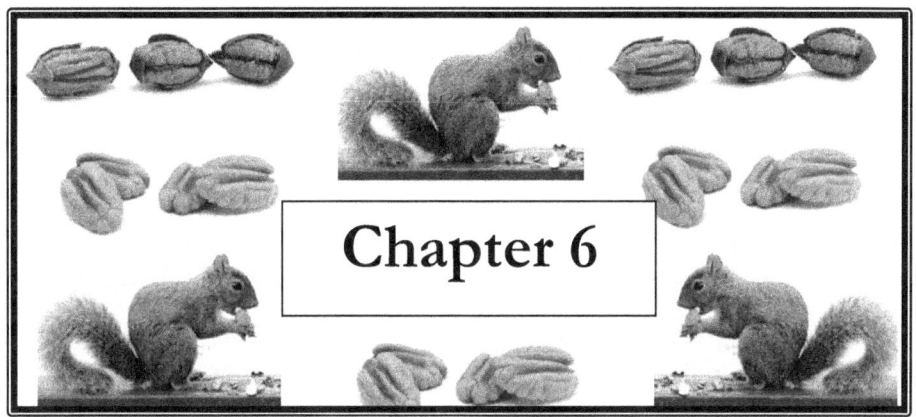

Pecans & Cancer Prevention

Pecans and Cancer Prevention- While much more basic research needs to be done, diet and weight control reduce risk for colorectal, prostate and breast cancers. Pecans are an excellent choice to reduce inflammation, to maintain a strong immune defense and a healthy population of helpful intestinal bacteria, and to avoid increased cell division that permits mutations that trigger uncontrolled cell growth. This chapter will summarize new knowledge about nuts and colon health, and will identify areas that need to be explored.

Inflammation Increases Likelihood of Colon Cancer- Inflammation causes overstimulation of the immune system, and in the long term correlates with cancer development in the colon and the liver. Chronic inflammation of the colon is called **colitis**, a painful inflammatory bowel disease in which the colon wall is swollen with fluid and infiltrated with immune cells. An overly refined diet with excess sugar, fat, and refined starches in prepared foods does not prevent inflammation, unlike whole foods including nuts.

The healthy colon is an absorptive organ for water, vitamins and minerals. It also contains a large number of *goblet cells* that secrete a protective barrier made of mucus and defensive, antibacterial proteins. Whereas the small intestine does not foster growth of microbes, the healthy colon contains an immense population of hundreds of different kinds of bacteria. To maintain a healthy barrier, a supply of fermentable carbohydrate (soluble dietary fiber), probiotics, and low environmental stress are required. Otherwise, harmful bacteria can multiply and create a harmful condition called **dysbiosis**. (**Figure 6.1**)

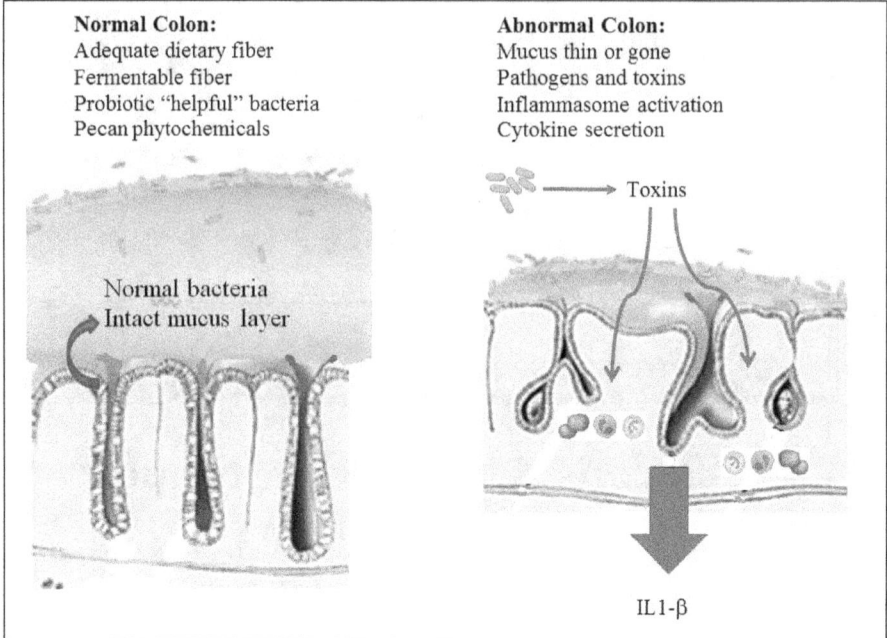

Normal Colon:
Adequate dietary fiber
Fermentable fiber
Probiotic "helpful" bacteria
Pecan phytochemicals

Normal bacteria
Intact mucus layer

Abnormal Colon:
Mucus thin or gone
Pathogens and toxins
Inflammasome activation
Cytokine secretion

Toxins

IL1-β

Figure 6.1. Normal, healthy colon (at left) compared to colon with bacterial overgrowth (dysbiosis), absence of the mucus barrier, chronic inflammation and cytokine secretion (left).

Dysbiosis and Cancer- The left side of **Figure 6.1** shows a healthy colon in which goblet cells actively produce a mucus barrier that keeps colon bacteria away from the colon tissue. A healthy bacteria population is maintained by adequate soluble dietary fiber and by the ability of phytochemicals from pecans and other foods and beverages to suppress growth of harmful pathogens. Soluble fiber is converted to *short chain fatty acids* that feed helpful bacteria. Immune cells are present in the tissue but there is little or no inflammation.

In contrast, an unhealthy colon loses its ability to secrete protective mucus, allowing bacteria and toxins to contact and invade the tissue and stimulate an immune reaction in the colon. The inflammasome system reacts to pathogens and toxins and secretes cytokines such as IL1-β that recruit other immune cells into the tissue (right side of **Figure 6.1**). Overstimulation of the immune system releases substances that damage the tissues, increase blood flow, and cause the colon tissue to swell painfully. As the colon attempts to repair itself, cell division is increased and the likelihood of acquiring mutations increases. These conditions favor cancer development.

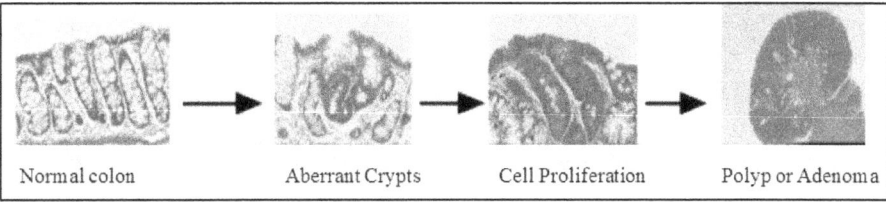

| Normal colon | Aberrant Crypts | Cell Proliferation | Polyp or Adenoma |

Figure 6.2. Mechanism of cancer requires multiple mutations over many years that convert normal tissue structure (example at left is colon) to abnormal structures with more rapidly dividing cells. As more mutations occur, growth increases until polyps or adenomas develop (right). These may be benign but further mutations make them malignant, and they invade other tissues.

Stages of Cancer Development- Nutritional prevention of cancer is difficult to study because tumors take many years to develop in humans and require multiple mutations (**Figure 6.2**). There are many individual steps in the overall process of DNA mutation, tumor initiation, progression, metastasis and immune defense.

Epidemiological Evidence- Vegetarian diets, increased physical activity, and maintenance of healthy weight reduce the risk of developing colon, breast and prostate cancer, whereas meat consumption increases the risk [68]. All public and private cancer advisory groups recommend increased consumption of cruciferous vegetables, fruits, and other whole foods including nuts.

It is possible but not proven that high nut consumption may reduce risk of colorectal cancer in women. A statistically significant reduction in risk was seen in the European Prospective Investigation into Cancer and Nutrition (EPIC) for women who consumed more than 6.2 grams of nuts per day [69]. This is a very low level of nut consumption, and no such result was seen in men at the same level of consumption. The result may depend on a gender difference such as sex steroids or responses to phytoestrogens, or perhaps a higher nut intake compared to body mass.

A study from Taiwan showed that peanut consumption is associated with reduced risk for colon cancer, and the effect in this study was also somewhat greater in women than in men [70]. To our knowledge, the Taiwanese study and the European study are the only ones that have made any preventative association between nuts and any cancer in people. No study has yet evaluated whether nut phytochemicals have a preventative effect. Nuts are good sources of phytoestrogens called enterolignans [10], so this potential gender difference deserves more research.

Preclinical Studies- There are numerous animal models of cancer. Usually the animals are fed a particular diet and then are exposed to a carcinogen that produces precancerous changes in cells. One study evaluated almond meal for the ability to reduce abnormal cell growth in laboratory rodents. Almond meal significantly reduced the number of precancerous, aberrant crypt foci 26 weeks after treatment with a carcinogen that produces colon cancer [71]. The mechanism may be an increase in molecular signals that block cancer initiation [72]. At present, there is no similar work based on other nuts, and no evidence that the same kind of events happen in people.

Anti-Cancer Phytonutrients- Pecans contain folate, vitamin E, selenium (an antioxidant trace element needed for antioxidant enzymes), oleic acid (a monounsaturated fat), proanthocyanidins, quercetin and ellagic acid, which all have anti-cancer properties. People who consume nuts tend also to increase folate consumption [73].

The Mediterranean diet is high in oleic acid as a result of emphasizing olive oil, and olive oil has been reported to have anti-cancer effects [74-76]. However, in addition to possible effects of oleic acid on gene expression [76], virgin olive oil contains several phenolic antioxidants that may have a more important effect on cancer risk [77, 78]. The protective antioxidants give olive oil its green color and unique flavor.

Pecan Bioactives and Cancer Prevention- Pecans contain quercetin, epigallocatechin gallate (EGCG), and proanthocyanidins. Each of these compounds or classes has been shown to prevent aspects of tumor development in laboratory animals and cell culture. Quercetin and EGCG are active in a variety of cancer models [79, 80]. Proanthocyanidins from a variety of sources are being evaluated for anti-cancer activity [81-83].

Multiple preclinical studies have shown that ellagic acid and ellagitannins from berries (but also present in pecans) prevent cancer development in animals. In particular, blackberries, black raspberries, and pomegranates are good sources of the protective compounds [84-86].

The flavonoid, quercetin, has been implicated in prevention of colon cancer, breast cancer and prostate cancer [84, 87, 88]. As with ellagic acid, berries are a good natural source. Pecans contain quercetin, so there is potential for cancer risk reduction.

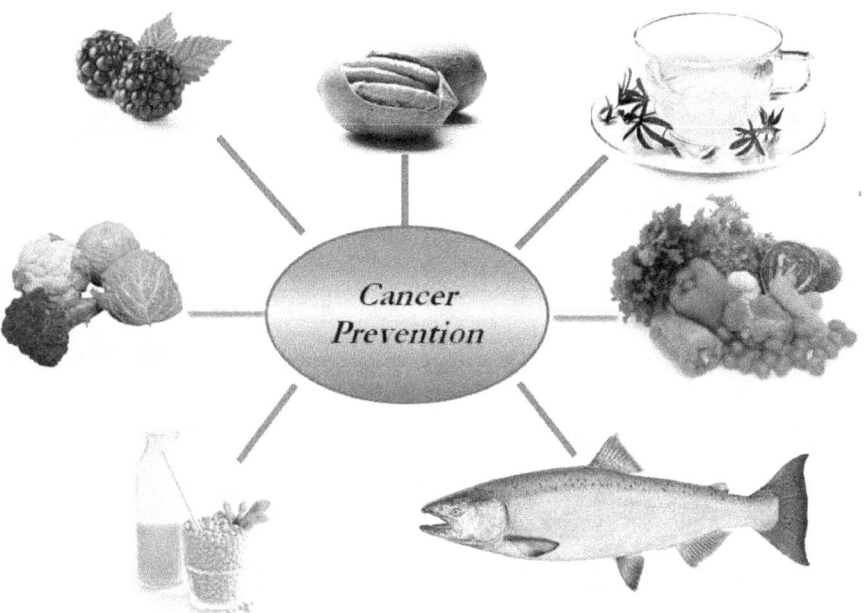

Figure 6.3- Elements of a cancer-preventing diet include nuts for healthy fats, vitamin E and selenium, green tea for catechins (EGCG), vegetables for carotenoids and flavonoids, salmon for omega-3 fatty acids, soy products for phytoestrogens, crucifers for compounds that increase detoxifying enzymes, and berries for ellagic acid and ellagitannins.

EGCG shows promise for prevention of colorectal cancer, prostate cancer and liver cancer [89, 90]. The major dietary source of EGCG is green tea, and regular consumption could be one reason that Asian dietary patterns tend to have lower incidence of some cancers than Western patterns. **Figure 6.3** illustrates ideas for diet and cancer prevention that are consistent with advice from the National Cancer Institute.

Similarly, numerous preclinical and mechanistic studies are evaluating effects of PACs for prevention of cancer, with special emphasis on oral cancer [83, 91, 92]. A question being evaluated is whether the short chain compounds called oligomeric PACs are more effective than the long chain compounds. Oligomeric PACs are found in grapes, grape seed extract, and a pine bark extract called pycnogenol.

Because pecans contain all of these compounds, it is clear that they may enhance an overall diet that also includes berries, red grapes, green tea, cocoa, and other potential cancer preventatives.

Glucose Feeds Cancer- Cancer cells rely on glucose for most of their energy metabolism [93], so it may be useful that pecans provide most of their energy as unsaturated fats. Conditions such as pre-diabetes and diabetes lead to elevated blood glucose, which is thought to favor cancer development [94], whereas weight loss helps reduce risk of cancer in people who are overweight or obese.

Because high blood glucose favors cancer cell metabolism, numerous epidemiological studies have assessed the relationship between dietary fiber, meal glycemic index and daily glycemic load to kinds of cancer. In large studies, so far no effect has been reported [95-97]. .

Advice from the National Cancer Institute- The major link between nuts and cancer prevention is their content of vitamin E and selenium, which have reduced cancer risk in some studies. Because nuts are good sources of these nutrients, nuts should be included in a dietary plan that helps lower cancer risk.

Take-Home Messages about Pecans and Cancer- Optimal strategies for cancer prevention include eating nuts as part of a diet based primarily on whole, plant-based foods. It is important to be physically active and maintain body weight, and to avoid known risk factors such as tobacco smoking and obesity. The most constructive advice may be to maintain digestive health and focus on an anti-inflammatory diet and lifestyle in the short term in order to prevent or reduce risk for cancer in the long term. Pecans are one of the most anti-inflammatory nuts and deserve to be part of a daily plan for risk reduction.

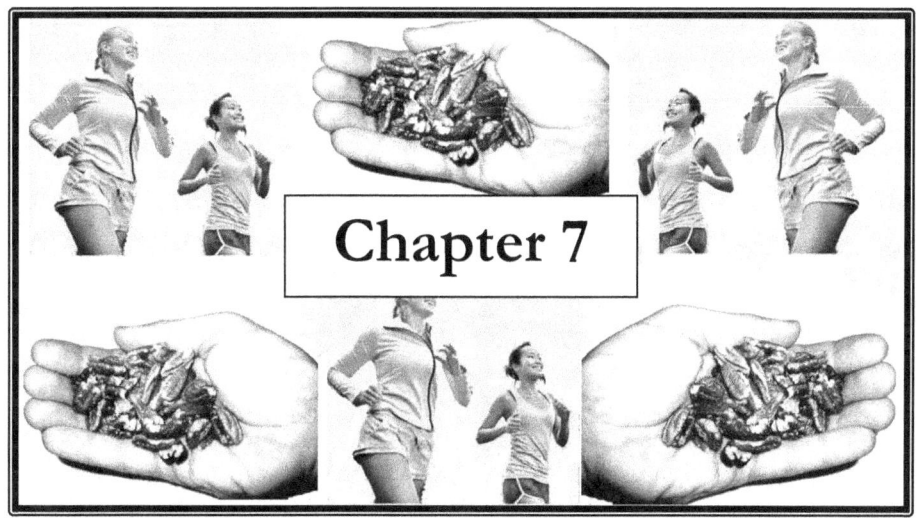

Pecans & Healthy Aging

Pecans for a Longer, Healthier Life- Scientific evidence is conclusive: smart dietary choices (including weekly nut consumption), risk avoidance, and useful physical activity can add ten years to your life [1]. Evidence suggests that human populations should be able to live to an average age of about 85 years, which would mean that fewer people would be dying in their 50's and more would live to be 100. Pecans are nutritional power choices because they provide an enriched source of phytochemicals, healthy fats, and minerals that help fight various chronic diseases.

The absolute maximum human lifespan is about 115 years, and there are advocates of life extension who think that this maximum could be increased. The jury is out on that question. We agree with Dr. Andrew Weil that nuts add more healthy years to your existing life. Scientists refer to the idea of adding more healthy years to your life by the awkward phrase, "compression of morbidity." This is not the same as extending the maximum lifespan, but the result is more healthy years of life.

Pecans improve the health of every major part of the body, from the brain to blood vessels, the heart, liver and gastrointestinal tract, with a very simple rule: People who eat pecans reap the benefits, others do not. Here is why.

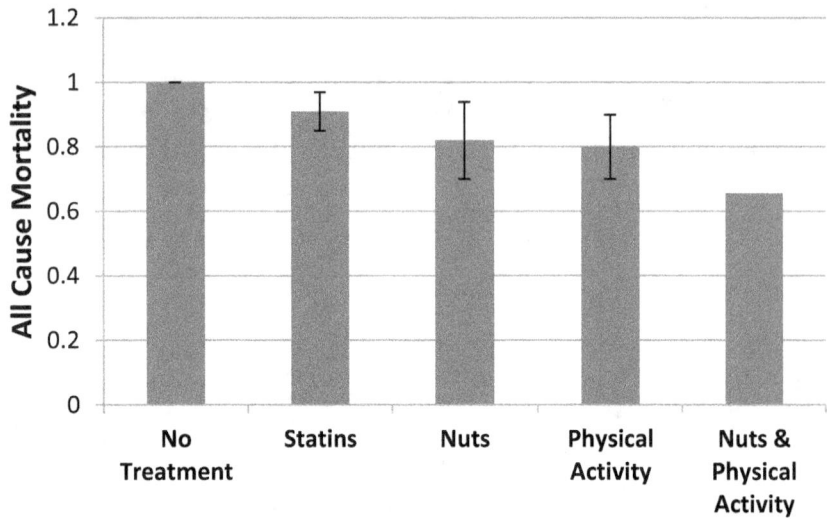

Figure 7.1. Effects of statin therapy, nut consumption, and physical activity on all-cause mortality for healthy people. Risk reduction is greater in all cases for people who already have coronary heart disease. Data from references [98-100].

Pecans Beat Statins at Adding Years of Life for Healthy People- The multi-billion dollar statin drug industry is pushing the boundaries of medicine. Originally, statins were prescribed for people with total cholesterol values over 240 mg/dL of blood plasma. Presently, the cut-off is 200 mg/dL, and there is a push to include adolescents and even otherwise healthy people at an average cost of $70 per month. A recent review found that statin therapy could reduce all-cause mortality in healthy people to 0.91, where 1.0 is average. Wow, 9%.

Regular nut consumption of 4-5 servings per week significantly decreases risk of dying even *more than statin drug therapy for healthy people* (**Figure 7.1**)[98-100]. The benefit of nut consumption is comparable to getting regular physical activity, and combining nuts and physical activity gives a lower risk [98]. And pecans nourish the muscles and brain, whereas statins cause neuromuscular toxicity and, in some people, transient amnesia-a sign of brain toxicity.

Pecan Therapy- Eating 4-5 servings of nuts per week reduces all-cause mortality about 20% to about 0.8 in healthy people. And you can't put statin drugs on pumpkin pie, statins just don't go well with vanilla ice cream. Yes, whole nuts are a bit expensive as foods go, but the serving size is small. Statin therapy for a family of four would cost around $300 a month, pecan "therapy" might run $30. A healthy diet is a whole lot less expensive than lifelong drug treatment or open-heart surgery.

The conclusion for healthy people is simple: Let's run and get some nuts!

Nuts for Reduced Stress Responses- We mentioned that regular nut consumption helps maintain normal blood pressure. One of the ways this happens is that blood pressure does not react as much to stress. To test effects of nut consumption on blood pressure, West and others [101] fed one or two servings of nuts per day for four weeks. They then measured changes in blood pressure while the subjects were performing math tests, and also tested their response to cold exposure. These tests increase blood pressure, heart rate, and cardiac output. However, subjects consuming nuts had less of a stress response. Systolic blood pressure did not increase as much as it did for subjects who were not eating nuts, and two servings per day gave the greatest reduction in a measure called total peripheral resistance (having less resistance usually means blood pressure is lower).

Pecans versus the Resveratrol Craze- A few years ago, scientists discovered that a phytochemical called resveratrol increases lifespan in fruit flies and some lower organisms, apparently by activating a gene called SIRT-1 [102]. Resveratrol is best known as being present in red wines (although at microgram levels) and possibly explaining why the French can eat high fat diets and not be affected by heart disease.

Naturally, it is now possible to buy dietary supplements, foods and beverages that are spiked with resveratrol (usually obtained from the root of Japanese Knotweed). Such supplements are always expensive compared to whole foods, and there is no evidence of long-term benefits in people.

Two points need to be made about the resveratrol craze. Firstly, the original work showed that other flavonoids that are much more abundant in foods (including pecans) also activate SIRT-1. Secondly, almost no one in nutritional research believes that taking a single, purified food supplement can duplicate the effect of eating whole foods.

Perhaps it has escaped people's attention that the French regularly eat nuts as part of their high-fat diets, but "The French Nut Paradox" has just not caught on yet.

Brain Benefits of Eating Whole Foods- Dr. James Joseph has made the point that whole foods beat supplements for brain health. His group found that eating blueberries slowed several measures of brain aging in rodents, and the benefit was apparently due to specific phytochemicals working in several brain areas [103, 104]. However, when the same studies were done with purified blueberry phytochemicals, the benefits were not seen. There was no individual phytochemical fraction or combination that duplicated the effect of eating the whole berries [105]. So much for pills.

Pecans as Nutrient-Rich Whole Foods that Nourish the Brain- There are approximately 47 essential nutrients, including 14 vitamins, 12 amino acids, 4 essential fatty acids, and 17 mineral elements in pecans. There are dozens more potential nutrients that may have health benefits but are under-studied, and then there are hundreds of non-nutritive but functional phytochemicals. To cite just two examples of nutrients that are important for brain health and aging, tree nuts contain sphingolipids [7], which are needed by the brain for normal function. Another kind of nut constituent called polyamine is necessary for normal health but declines with aging [106].

It is clear that fat-soluble antioxidants are good for the brain, partly because nerve cells contain large amounts of lipids that must be protected against damage by free radicals. It is interesting that pecans, walnuts and pistachios have very high levels of an antioxidant called gamma-tocopherol, whereas almonds and hazelnuts contain primarily alpha-tocopherol [107]. Including pecans in weekly meals will make sure that adequate amounts of this unique, fat-soluble antioxidant are available for brain health.

There is an old saying that fish are good brain food. It is good news that the same may be said of pecans!

It should be obvious that all of these compounds will never be studied one at a time, much less in all possible combinations. Perhaps it is enough to know that eating whole nuts is good for the whole body throughout the lifespan. Current evidence and common sense tell us that there are many smart choices, and eating more nuts is one that fits every known cuisine and dietary pattern.

How much should I eat? Average nut consumption in the United States is currently half a serving per week and the recommendation is 4-5 servings per week. The situation is even more dramatic, because peanut butter counts as a serving. Peanuts are legumes. We think evidence suggests that 4-5 servings of tree nuts each week produces the biggest health benefit for the 98% of people who are not allergic to nuts.

Pecans Put the "Nut" in Nutrition- Part of the improvement in heart health with nut consumption is due to their healthy fats, low glycemic index, high fiber, vitamin E, and useful mineral balance. That said, pecans and other nuts contain nutrients whose benefits have not been fully explored yet.

In this light, pecans contain coenzyme Q10, which is necessary for energy metabolism in the heart and in the brain. This coenzyme is not considered essential because it is made in the body, but there may be times when it is limited. For example, statin drugs block the production of CoQ10, which may explain part of their neuromuscular toxicity.

Pecans contain a combination of nutrients that maintain normal fat metabolism in the liver. Imbalanced nutrition and too much abdominal fat can cause accumulation of fat in the liver, which is an inflammatory condition called Non-Alcoholic Fatty Liver Disease. Nuts are good sources of vitamins and vitamin-like compounds that help mobilize this fat and maintain health [108].

Pecans contain a variety of trace minerals that support bone health and may slow the development of osteoporosis. In some cases, the functions are well known, in other cases, knowledge is limited. For example, nuts are a good source of the element, boron, which may be important for bone health, but the reason has not been identified [109].

Nuts are a good source of mineral elements including chromium, barium, copper, iron, lithium, magnesium, manganese, nickel, zinc and potassium, but are very low in sodium (in this case, being low is good). Needless to say, these minerals have hundreds of biochemical functions, and it is a very good idea for eating whole foods like pecans that provide a great balance.

Pecans contain inositol, which has numerous metabolic functions. Even though it can be made in the body, pecans are a good source of this compound.

The brain contains complex lipids, most of which are known only to specialists. Pecans contain building blocks for most of these lipids, which may be beneficial in slowing age-related changes such as Parkinsonism and Alzheimer's Disease [110-112]. There is also evidence that lipids called phytosterols in pecans and walnuts can block the formation of Alzheimer's plaque by blocking a deposit called amyloid [112-114].

This book is about health benefits of pecans, but evidence is strongest for nuts in general. Given that it would be helpful for low nut consumers to increase their consumption by ten-fold, there is room for all the common nuts. It is fine to mix it up with pecans, walnuts, almonds, cashews, pistachios, and Brazil nuts as you prefer.

Calorie Restriction, Gene Expression and Brain Aging- A proven way to extend life in laboratory rodents is by reducing calorie intake while maintaining normal intakes of essential amino acids, fatty acids, vitamins and minerals [115-

119]. It is not clear that the same thing is true for humans, and recent work with Rhesus monkeys found no effect on all-cause mortality by reducing calorie intake by 10-30%.

Calorie restriction tends to decrease the activity of the stress related genes [120-122]. This happens in just about every organ that has been tested, from muscle to liver to brain. So one of the theories of how calorie restriction extends life is that it helps protect the brain against age-related injury. If nerve cells die, they usually can't be replaced, so it is very good news that we might be able to protect them. One of the theories is that aging increases oxidative stress and decreases our ability to combat it. Calorie restriction seems to boost the brains defenses while reducing the accumulation of tiny daily injuries.

Nuts, Berries, Leafy Greens and Brain Aging-Brain aging is not just due to oxygen free radicals. Inflammation, release of calcium from dying cells, and bleeding from tiny capillaries are other causes of brain aging. But there is good news. A dramatic breakthrough was found when animals were fed diets high in phytophenolics from grapes, blueberries, strawberries, spinach or kale [123-125].

When animals were fed a diet that contained 1-2% dried blueberries, strawberries, or spinach, the blueberry fed animals maintained their coordination and cognitive function significantly longer than animals that only got rodent chow [103]. The berries had the most beneficial effect, and when this news was reported in the popular press, the price of blueberries skyrocketed. Spinach also is protective, and grape seed extract rejuvenates brain antioxidant defenses [126].

One effect of consuming pecan power phytochemicals is altered gene expression in organs such as liver and brain [127]. Adaptive changes in gene expression help defend the body against the ill effects of aging.

Plant Polyphenols and Life Extension- It turns out that overfeeding increases stress-associated genes in brain and other tissues, whereas consuming a highly nutritious diet that is restricted in calories decreases the activity of stress related genes [128, 129]. What has come as a surprise that plant polyphenols like resveratrol can increase lifespan even in animals that overeat. There is hope for people who prefer to eat normal portions!

Several phytochemicals improve DNA repair by a pathway that is found in humans and it has already been shown that low concentrations of resveratrol activate a pathway that increases lifespan in human cells [102, 130, 131].

Because DNA repair is improved, the cells do not collect mutations and become cancerous as rapidly as they do in the absence of resveratrol.

The same compounds also promote mobilization of fat from fat cells [132]. Another effect is to improve insulin sensitivity [133], and it is known that becoming fat decreases insulin sensitivity and raises blood glucose towards the diabetic range. The result is that pecan constituents including proanthocyanidins and quercetin have many beneficial effects on our metabolism. They are a power choice in the "phyte" for better health and life extension.

Pecans and Extension of Your Love Life- In both men and women, pecan phytochemicals improve blood vessel health in a variety of ways, and that benefits the health of all organs [134]. Because nut consumption lowers cholesterol and reduces cholesterol oxidation, blood vessel health is improved not only in the heart but also in ways that help prevent erectile dysfunction. In addition, proanthocyanidins, ellagic acid, quercetin and other flavonoids increase production of nitric oxide, which relaxes blood vessels and improves blood flow [135]. Sometimes called a "co-morbidity," an impaired sexual response frequently arises when a person develops heart disease, diabetes, or serious obesity. Nuts also contribute through their arginine content because arginine is the compound needed for the body to make nitric oxide to relax blood vessels and increase blood flow.

Another way that flavonoids from nuts, berries, fruits and vegetables improve blood flow is by inhibiting an enzyme in the blood vessel wall called phosphodiesterase E5 [136]. Inhibitors of this enzyme are used in medicine under the trade names of Viagra®, Cialis®, and Levitra®. Along with other rich sources of these compounds, pecans can help prevent long term damage to blood vessels and nerves needed for a sexual response, as well as helping provide good blood flow in the short term after meals that provide these important phytochemicals. Beyond blood flow, a new report suggests that nut consumption improves semen vitality in men who consume Western-style diets [137]. Perhaps a recipe for pecan-encrusted oysters would be useful!

Pecan Polyphenolics "Phyte" for Health- As we get older, the chromosomes that contain our genes progressively shorten and lose a protective cap on each end. The ends get chewed off by an enzyme called telomerase. It would be useful to block the enzyme so cells could continue dividing in a healthy manner. Early tests concerning whether polyphenols affect the telomerase enzyme have been encouraging. The catechins in tea (especially green tea) do inhibit telomerase, and this has been suggested as one reason

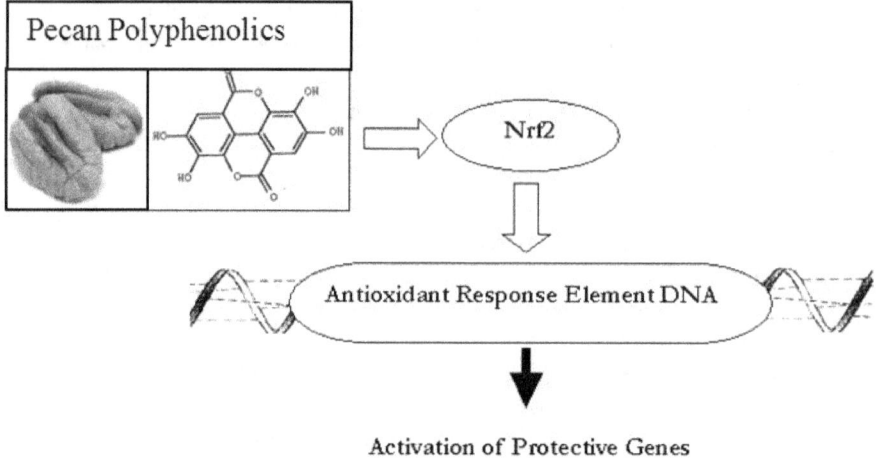

Figure 7.2. Pecan phytochemicals such as ellagic acid change gene activity. One example is the ability to activate a gene controller called Nrf2, which activates the Antioxidant Response Element in DNA. Activating this element activates production of a variety of proteins that protect cells against damage by free radicals and decrease production of inflammatory gene products.

catechins have anti-cancer effects [138]. Pecans also have catechins, and we are optimistic that pecan extracts can be shown to inhibit telomerase.

What you should know about genes and health- Most people know that they inherit their genes from their parents, but may think that there is nothing a person can do to modify gene function. Not so! Your diet and daily activities are the most powerful ways you can help your genes keep you healthy. But the activity of your genes is responsive to good nutrients, energy intake, sunshine, fresh air, healthy activity, and a good mood. Gene activity also responds to overeating, smog, refined foods, pollution, lack of activity, and feeling lousy! People who make good choices about their diets, family life, choices of occupation and leisure activities really are affecting their genes and their health.

Pecan phytochemicals affect genes that keep every part of the body healthy- It is fairly easy to understand how phytonutrients in pecans can improve the health of the gastrointestinal tract. After all, eating pecans is a way of delivering these good chemicals to every part of the bowel. And it is not too hard to see how they could also affect the blood vessels to lower the incidence of heart disease. Once the phytonutrients are absorbed, they go into circulation in the blood, and some of them are carried on the same particles that move cholesterol around the body. Their antioxidant function prevents cholesterol from being even more damaging to the walls of blood vessels.

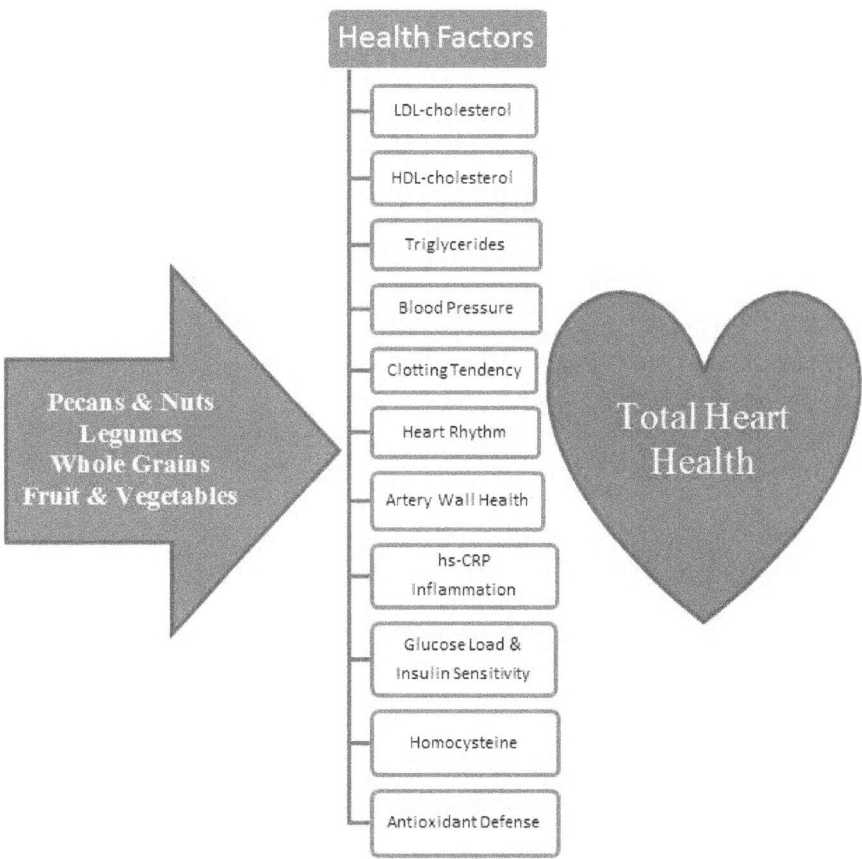

Figure 7.3. Pecan consumption as part of a healthy diet affects more than a dozen factors in that affect health of the heart, brain, blood vessels, and blood clotting mechanisms.

Pecans for an Ounce of Prevention- Earlier chapters in this book explain some of the beneficial effects of pecan phytochemicals on the heart and blood vessels, and how they defend against free radicals, reduce inflammatory diseases and may even prevent some cancers. **Figure 7.3** summarizes several of these points. Because having healthy blood vessels and healthy blood pressure affects the entire body, these benefits manifest themselves as better health for the whole person—and that is the desired outcome.

In every case, there is published, scientific evidence to back up these health benefits that can be obtained without buying expensive food supplements. All you need to do is add pecans to your shopping list every month, if you are not already doing this.

People who eat foods that help defend their blood vessels and cardiovascular systems tend to stay healthy longer and not suffer from premature heart disease. Pecan phytochemicals are good for the heart and blood vessels. Pecans fit in well with a heart healthy diet, and that includes helping keep the blood pressure down, too. People who protect themselves from early heart disease and stroke are protecting themselves against conditions that account for nearly half of all deaths.

Pecans are whole foods that have healing, anti-inflammatory qualities. To benefit, it goes without saying that pecans and other nuts should be consumed as a regular part of family meals. Let us take a break from the science. The final chapter will give some ideas about using pecans to prepare delicious meals.

Pecan Power in Your Diet

Pecans Boost Meals in a Flash- There is strong and convincing evidence that regular nut consumption increases nutritional quality of meals, decreases heart disease, and increases longevity. The first seven chapters of this book summarize the evidence for health benefits. Knowing about this in theory is good, but how much better is it to eat pecans regularly and put this information to use!

It is easy to incorporate pecans into your daily diet whether or not you are a cook. Let's consider a person who cooks skillfully and can keep pecans on hand for daily incorporation into the diet. Though thousands of recipes are available for pecans (see ideas and links in this chapter), we suggest that in order to get a significant amount of pecans into meals, the cook should exercise some culinary license and double or triple the amount of pecans and use them for garnishing as well. Many recipes are unduly timid and could use the nutritional boost that extra pecans provide. Remember, the goal is to eat at least one ounce of nuts a day.

Now let's take the second situation for a person who does little "from scratch" cooking, but still wants to incorporate nuts into the daily diet. This is extremely simple and requires only buying a large bag of pecans to have on hand to add to prepared foods, take-out foods, salads, desserts and snacks. This is so much easier than putting them into recipes, because you simply add them to your meals or use them to replace unhealthful snacks and to make convenience foods more healthful. In this type of kitchen, the best place to have a bag of pecans is right next to the microwave. A second place is in the refrigerator with the salad items.

Many Americans purchase frozen entrees to save time for weekday breakfast, lunch and supper. After long days at work, we just don't always have time or energy to prepare family meals from scratch. A simple way to boost the nutritional quality of prepared foods is to add a handful of pecans or other nuts just before serving.

Pecan Versatility- Pecans are excellent raw or toasted, and combine very well with berries, fruits, nut breads, entrees, salads and desserts. After all, if your plan includes improving heart health and adding ten years to your life, why not aim for the best quality of life you can achieve? Along with berries, fruit, whole grains and dark green salad vegetables, pecans help add nutritional power to every diet. Adding pecans makes dishes more nutritious, more healing, and anti-inflammatory. Increasing longevity never tasted so good!

Top Pecan Recipe Sources

National Pecan Shellers Association-Recipes
http://www.ilovepecans.org/nutrition.html
Georgia Pecan Commission-Recipes
http://www.georgiapecans.org/
Texas Pecan Growers Association-Recipes
http://www.tpga.org/activities.php
NutHealth.org-Recipes
http://www.nuthealth.org/pecans/
Nuts for Life (Australian)-Recipes
www.nutsforlife.com

Pecans in a Healing Food Pyramid- The menu ideas presented in this chapter are based on the healing food guide shown in **Figure 8**.1, which includes nuts at the top of the pyramid. In contrast to this power choice, sugar, high fructose corn sweetener, and refined starches are not food groups. Because most traditional cooking, and especially Southern cooking, uses pecans primarily for sweetened desserts, we recommend substituting non-caloric sweeteners such as Splenda®* to keep the dishes healthful and healing.

*Splenda is a registered trademark of Tate & Lyle and McNeill Nutritionals LLC.

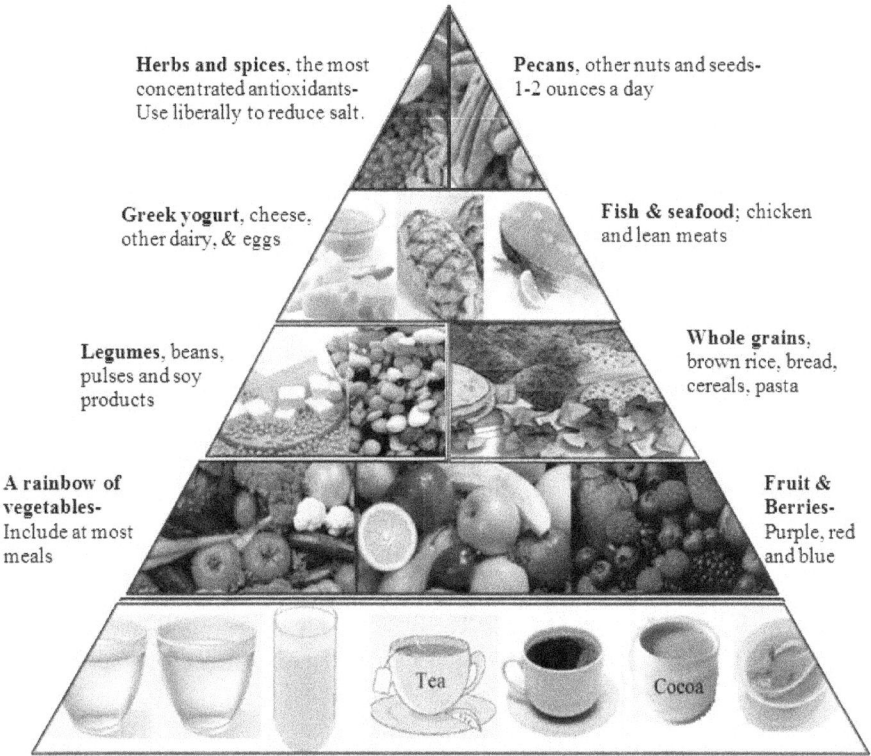

Herbs and spices, the most concentrated antioxidants- Use liberally to reduce salt.

Pecans, other nuts and seeds- 1-2 ounces a day

Greek yogurt, cheese, other dairy, & eggs

Fish & seafood; chicken and lean meats

Legumes, beans, pulses and soy products

Whole grains, brown rice, bread, cereals, pasta

A rainbow of vegetables- Include at most meals

Fruit & Berries- Purple, red and blue

Tea

Cocoa

Healing beverages include water, soy milk, teas, coffee, cocoa, soup broth, 100% fruit or vegetable juice, with reduced fat milk and wine on occasion. The proportions in the pyramid approximate amounts to include in daily and weekly meal plans.

Figure 8.1. A healing food guide shows general principles for using meals and beverages to reduce inflammation and allow tissues to heal on a daily basis. Pecans and other nuts are especially useful when they replace sugary or fatty snacks. These are indicated at the apex of the pyramid along with herbs and spices, which are the most concentrated sources of anti-inflammatory compounds in the diet. Balance of n-3 and n-6 fatty acids is ensured by eating fish and seafood twice a week, and by selecting healthful cooking oils for n-3 and monounsaturated fats.

The Healing Pyramid "from Soup to Nuts"- Notice the bottom tier of the pyramid is composed of liquids. Water intake is very important because keeping well hydrated and avoiding dehydration is essential for everyone. First of all, pure water is a refreshing beverage, although it lacks antioxidants. Other healthful beverages that do include antioxidants include soy milk, tea, herbal teas, coffee, cocoa (no sugar added) and soups. It is important that one

eliminate sodas and sugary drinks from the diet. For creamers, try substituting vanilla soy milk in coffees and teas if desired.

The next tier of the food pyramid is a high intake of a rainbow of vegetables and fruits. In the vegetable category, choose a range of vegetables from red, yellow, orange, green, purple, brown and white colors. In the fruit section, choose an array of colored fruits from the produce section. Finally, get berries from the fresh or frozen produce sections as the purple, red and blue range contains powerful phytochemicals for the diet.

The middle tier adds plant-based proteins to the diet with a wide array of legumes, beans, soy products and whole grain products as well as brown and black rice. After the diet has been composed of the bottom three tiers, it is time to add some healthy choices from animal-derived foods: Greek yogurt, cheeses, eggs, fish, seafood, chicken, turkey and very lean meats.

Finally, the top tier of the healing food pyramid also consists of natural real foods, including pecans. This top tier also includes the wide array of culinary herbs and spices. Like pecans, these culinary seasoning agents are very concentrated plant-based sources of phytochemicals that add greater health benefits to the diet.

For people who cook, many recipes are just wimpy when it comes to the amount of an herb or a spice to add to the recipe. One rule of thumb is that herbs and spices are acquired tastes. Most recipes may call for a small amount of a combination of herbs and spices, but remind the cook to "adjust" seasonings in the final stage of cooking. This is where one may divide a dish into low seasoning for the person who has not yet acquired a taste for herbs and spices, but may add more for those with palates favoring highly seasoned food.

For people who do not cook, adjusting seasonings to taste can be done for everything from breakfast cereals to convenience dinners. Anyone can turn a bland meal into a well-seasoned meal. Besides improving taste, one of the advantages of cultivating a palate preferring foods seasoned with herbs and spices is that it can significantly increase the health benefits of a given meal. It can also reduce the amount of salt in the diet. There is little need for adding salt to most whole foods that are seasoned with herbs and spices. Canned foods and prepared foods already contain a lot of salt. Use the top of the healing pyramid to reduce salt consumption without sacrificing enjoyment.

Pecans for Breakfast- Breakfasts are an easy place to incorporate pecans. COOK YES will put ground or chopped pecans in pancakes, waffles, muffins, breads, bread puddings or coffee cakes and incorporate whole or chopped pecans as the primary ingredient in toppings or spreads. COOK NO has it very easy. Pancakes, waffles, bagels or toast can be heated in microwave and pecans put on top with syrup or spread. Breakfast cereals will all benefit from a handful of pecans in the bowl.

Pecans for Quick Breakfasts and Snacks

Greek Yogurt (flavor of choice)
Add one handful of pecans
Half handful of dried berries or plums (prunes)

Breakfast Cereal (whole grain of choice)
Add one handful of pecans
Half handful of dried berries
Soy Milk (vanilla)

Desk Drawer Super Snack
1 large bag of pecans
1 large bag of dried berries
Dark chocolate pieces

Snacks are an excellent place to double up on the health value of pecans. If at home or office or school, a bag of pecans with a bag of dried berries (cran-raisins are excellent, also dried cherries, blueberries or plums) can be placed in a convenient spot for snacks to eliminate unhealthy sweet or starchy choices. At the office, reach for a handful of pecans/berries with morning coffee or tea. You get the benefit of the pecans, berries and coffee (the major source of plant antioxidants for most adult Americans!) while eliminating the donuts, chips, cookies and sodas from the diet. Don't eliminate snacks; just replace one convenient unhealthy temptation with an equally convenient, but healthy snack. Just keep pecans in your desk drawer at the office, book-bag at school or near the microwave or refrigerator at home. It helps to eliminate unhealthy snack items from your grocery cart and avoid the vending machine temptations when you get that hungry, hollow feeling. That mid-morning or mid-afternoon snack now becomes a low salt, low glycemic power choice in the overall diet.

Pecan-Banana Muffins

Ingredients

- 2 cups biscuit mix
- 4 overripe bananas
- 1/2 cup brown sugar or ¼ cup Splenda®
- 3/4 cup (1 1/2 sticks) unsalted butter, melted and cooled
- 2 eggs
- 1 teaspoon pure vanilla extract
- 2 teaspoons cinnamon
- 1 cup chopped pecans

Directions

Preheat oven to 375 degrees F and lightly butter 2 muffin tins (unless using foil muffin cups or a silicon baking sheet*).

Mash the bananas in a small bowl, then whip in brown sugar until well blended. Then add the melted butter, eggs, and vanilla. Beat well, scraping down the sides of the bowl once or twice. Mix in the dry ingredients just until incorporated. Fold in the nuts and spoon the batter into the muffin tins or silicone baking sheet to fill the cups about halfway.

Bake until a toothpick stuck in the muffins comes out clean, 18 to 20 minutes. Let cool for a few minutes before turning the muffins out. Serve warm or at room temperature.

*Silicone baking ware is non-stick and does not require butter or grease.

Adding more pecans to any recipe improves its nutritional, health-promoting value, so feel free to add more nuts according to your own knowledge and taste preferences.

Georgia Pork Tenderloins with Peaches and Pecans

- 1 pound of pork tenderloin cut into ¾ in slices

- 1 tablespoon olive oil

- 8 green onions, sliced on slant

- 4 cloves of garlic, minced

- ½ teaspoon cayenne pepper

- 1 can condensed golden mushroom soup

- 1 can (15 oz) sliced peaches (lite) , drained (reserve the juice)

- 2 tablespoons tamari sauce (or soy sauce)

- 2 tablespoons honey

- 2 cups toasted pecans

Heat oil in a 10 inch skillet over medium-high heat. Add pork medallions and cook until browned on both sides, then remove to a plate. In the same skillet, add the green onions and garlic and stir fry for 1 min. Then add cayenne pepper, the golden mushroom soup, the reserved peach juice, tamari or soy sauce and honey. Bring to a gentle boil and cook for about 5 min. Put browned pork medallions back into the skillet and the sliced peaches. Continue cooking until pork is cooked through and peaches are hot. Finally, add the toasted pecans and serve immediately with rice.

This recipe tastes great, with flavor and aromas arising from the surprising combination of onions, spices, and peaches that add sweetness and tenderness to the pork entrée.

Pecan-Crusted Baked Fish

Combine these ingredients or use a spice mixture of your choice:

> 6 tablespoons Italian seasoned fine bread crumbs
> 6 tablespoons finely chopped pecans (enough to fill a small coffee grinder)
> 1/4 teaspoon Creole or Italian seasoning
> 1/4 teaspoon garlic powder
> 1/4 teaspoon onion powder
> 1/4 teaspoon ground black pepper

Beat two eggs with one cup of olive oil

Cut 1-2 pounds of any white fish, salmon or your favorite fish fillets into servings and dredge in the egg mixture.

Coat fillets in the pecan mixture.

Place in a baking dish coated with olive oil.

Bake at 400 degrees F for 15-20 minutes or until fish flakes easily with a fork.

Remove from oven and drizzle with fresh lemon if desired.

Serve with your choice of side dishes. It was great with a leafy green salad and rosemary baked potatoes.

We made this entree with fresh Gulf redfish. It was excellent! All marine fish are good sources of omega-3 fatty acids (DHA and EPA), and salmon are excellent sources. Combining pecans and fresh fish makes this the best for taste and heart health.

Pecan, Apple & Cranberry Field Greens with Vinaigrette

Ingredients:

- 3 cups diced cooked chicken
- 1/2 cup dried cranberries
- 1/2 cup diced celery
- 1/4 cup finely chopped red onion
- 1 cup diced apple
- 1 cup chopped or whole pecans
- 4 tablespoons olive oil mayonnaise
- 1 tablespoon lemon juice
- 1/2 – 1 teaspoon curry powder (to taste)
- 1/4 teaspoon ground black pepper
- Bed of field green lettuce mixture per serving

Combine the chicken, cranberries, celery, onion, apple, and pecans.

In a cup or small bowl combine the mayonnaise, lemon juice, curry powder and pepper. Stir into the chicken, adding more mayonnaise as needed and for taste. Serve the chicken salad mixture on a bed of field greens.

Pecans work splendidly to complement berries and a variety of fruit. You can use this recipe or wing it and make up your own with the ingredients in your refrigerator. Your family will be benefitting from all the major classes of phytochemicals found in the Healing Foods Pyramid.

Pecan-Smothered Sweet Potato Soufflé

Ingredients

> 3 cup mashed sweet potatoes*
> 1/2 teaspoon salt
> 1 cup sugar
> 2 eggs
> 1/2 cup milk
> 1/3 cup melted butter

Mix ingredients and beat well. Pour into a well-greased baking dish. Mix topping (below).

Pecan Topping

> 1/2 cup plain flour
> 1/3 cup melted butter
> 1/2 cup brown sugar or ¼ cup Splenda®
> 1 cup chopped pecans

Mix ingredients and spread on top of soufflé mixture.
Bake at 350 degrees F for 30 minutes.

*Prepare from 2-3 fresh sweet potatoes or use instant mashed sweet potatoes that are available in grocery stores.

This scrumptious dish has many possible variations, and combines the nutritional power of two foods, pecans and sweet potatoes.

Keeping in mind the fact that great food is the least expensive way to manage your health, more recipes are suggested on the following pages.

Pecan & Wild Rice & Quinoa Pilaf

Ingredients:

> 1 tablespoon olive oil
> 1/3 cup finely chopped onion
> 1/3 cup finely chopped celery
> 1 cup chopped pecans
> 1 cup quinoa, rinsed and drained
> 3 cups chicken broth or vegetable stock
> 1 cup cooked wild rice

1. Heat oil in large saucepan at medium temperature. Sauté onion and celery for 5 minutes until onions are clear.
2. Stir in pecans and quinoa and cook for 2 more minutes.
3. Add the chicken broth and bring to a boil. Reduce heat to low, cover, and simmer for about 20 minutes.
4. Stir in wild rice, cover, and simmer for 2-3 minutes.
5. Season to taste

Spicy Pecan Movie Treats

Ingredients:

> 4 cups pecan halves
> 3 tablespoons butter
> 5 tablespoons granular Splenda®
> ½ teaspoon cayenne pepper
> 2 tablespoons cinnamon
> 1 teaspoon salt or salt substitute

Melt butter over medium heat in a non-stick large skillet. Add the whole pecans, Splenda®, cinnamon, cayenne and salt. Stir constantly for about 3 minutes or until pecans start to brown. Remove from heat and turn onto a glass plate or a cookie sheet until cool.

Pecan & Havarti Quesadillas

Sprinkle 1 side of an 8-inch soft flour tortilla with 1/3 cup (1 1/2 oz.) shredded Havarti cheese and 2 tablespoons chopped toasted pecans.

Fold in half over filling. Heat quesadilla in a lightly greased skillet over medium-high heat 2 minutes on each side or until cheese melts and tortilla is golden brown.

Cut into wedges, and serve with slices of ripe pears or apples.

Pecan & Chicken Salad or Sandwich

Ingredients:
>   2 cups of cooked, diced chicken breast
>   1/4 to 1/2 cup of mayonnaise
>   1 tablespoons orange juice frozen concentrate
>   1 cup of whole toasted pecans; measure then crush or chop
>   ½ cup dried cranberries
>   6 mandarin oranges pieces (optional)
>   Salt and pepper
>   Green leaf lettuce
>   Bread of choice

Start by toasting whole pecans at 350 degrees F for about 5 minutes. Measure 1 cup of whole pecans, then chop to desired size.

Combine cooked chicken, mayo, orange juice concentrate, chopped pecans, cranberries and mandarin oranges (if desired) in a medium-sized bowl. Add salt and pepper to taste. Make sandwich with the spread and a leaf of lettuce. Or, serve the salad in a mound on a bed of lettuce.

Elegant Spicy Pecan Pumpkin Pie

Ingredients

     1 unbaked deep-dish (10") pie pastry
     1 (30 oz) can of pumpkin pie mix
     2/3 cups of evaporated milk
     3 eggs, lightly beaten
     1 tablespoon additional pumpkin pie spice (optional, but good)
     ¾ cups coarsely chopped pecans
     1 cup of whole pecans (enough to create top design)

1. Preheat oven to 425 degrees F.
2. Spread the chopped pecans onto the deep-dish pie shell
3. Combine pumpkin pie mix, evaporated milk, beaten eggs and the pumpkin pie spice in a large bowl; mix well. Pour on top of the chopped pecans in the prepared pie shell.
4. Bake for 15-20 minutes at 425 degrees F until pie is set. Then remove from oven and place whole pecans on top of the pie in a circular array pattern starting at the center and working toward the edges.
5. Reduce temperature to 350 degrees F and continue baking for 50-60 minutes until the center of pie is set and edges are brown. (Check with a toothpick without disturbing pecan design).
6. Remove from oven and allow to rest 30 min. Serve hot or cold. Delicious with or without ice cream or whipped cream topping.

Concluding Thoughts- The first seven chapters of this book describe the scientific evidence that shows pecans and other nuts can add years to your life. People who eat several servings of nuts a week improve the nutritional quality of their diets, and as a result have better heart health, better immune function, and better cognitive abilities. To derive these benefits and get the phytochemical power, the first step is to buy an ample supply from your market so they are available at home. Then add them to your recipes, or ones mentioned in this chapter. You can be confident knowing that people who eat pecans get more enjoyment from their meals and complete nutrition that really goes "from soup to nuts"!

Biomedical References Cited in the Text

For a complete list of the scientific publications cited in this work, please refer to our web page dedicated to the health benefits of pecans:

www.pecanhealth.com

Biographical Sketches of the Authors

James L. Hargrove, Ph.D. is an emeritus Associate Professor in the Department of Foods and Nutrition at the University of Georgia. He earned a B.S. in Biology, M.S. in Physiology, and a Ph.D. in Biology and Physiology from Utah State University. He did research at the University of Iowa Diabetes Center befo

re taking a faculty position at Emory University School of Medicine. Currently, Dr. Hargrove is director of a Nutraceutical Research Laboratory in the Dept. of Foods and Nutrition at The University of Georgia, Athens, GA. He develops new nutraceutical products, trains graduate students and teaches both undergraduate and graduate students in nutrition science. Dr. Hargrove is the author of several books related to nutrient control of gene expression and computer modeling in nutrition. He has published over 100 research papers, books, book chapters, and conference papers.

Diane K. Hartle, Ph.D. earned a B.S. in Biochemistry from the University of Minnesota and a Ph.D. in Pharmacology from the University of Iowa. She has had faculty appointments at Emory University in Atlanta, GA and The University of Georgia in Athens, GA. Currently Dr. Hartle is an emerita Associate Professor and Director of a Nutraceutical Research Laboratory in the College of Pharmacy at the University of Georgia. She is a member of the Graduate Faculty and trains graduate students in biomedical research. Besides conducting and publishing nutraceutical research, she studies natural products and health, and teaches pharmacology and nutraceutical science to Pharm.D. students and graduate students in health-related Ph.D. programs.

Phillip Greenspan, Ph.D. earned an A.B. from Rutgers College and a Ph.D. from the University of Iowa in Pharmacology. He has had academic appointments at Bowman Gray School of Medicine and the University of South Carolina School of Medicine. Dr. Greenspan is an Associate Professor in the College of Pharmacy at the University of Georgia. He is Director of a Nutraceutical Research Laboratory developing new nutraceutical products and trains graduate students in the Department of Pharmaceutical and Biomedical Sciences. He teaches physiology and pharmacology to Pharm.D. and graduate students in various health-related Ph.D. programs.